IMPERFECT HEART

STORIES OF MYOCARDIAL BRIDGES

This book reveals a solution for your unexplained heart attack-like symptoms—chest pain, shortness of breath, pain in the neck, back, or jaw. It's not just stress. Something's wrong. There's hope.

JEFF HOLDEN

Adapted from original interviews on the podcast "Imperfect Heart".

Copyright and Release of Liability

Copyright © 2025 NewSense Strategies, Inc.

All rights reserved. No part of this publication may be reproduced, distributed, or transmitted in any form or by any means, including photocopying, recording, or other electronic or mechanical methods, without the prior written permission of the author, except in the case of brief quotations embodied in critical reviews and certain other noncommercial uses permitted by copyright law. For permission requests, contact the author at jeff@hearmenowstudio.com.

The information contained in this book is for educational and informational purposes only and is provided "as is." The author and publisher make no representations or warranties of any kind, express or implied, about the completeness, accuracy, reliability, suitability, or availability of the information contained herein. Any reliance you place on such information is strictly at your own risk.

To the fullest extent permitted by law, the author and publisher disclaim all liability for any losses, injuries, or damages resulting from the use or misuse of this book. This book is not intended as a substitute for professional advice. Always seek the guidance of a qualified professional regarding any questions or concerns you may have related to the topics covered.

By reading this book, you acknowledge and agree that the author and publisher are not responsible for any outcomes, financial losses, health implications or other consequences resulting from your use of the information contained within.

For additional information or inquiries, please contact:

Jeff Holden, NewSense Strategies, Inc. dba Hear Me Now Studio, 7921 Kingswood Drive, Ste. A1, Citrus Heights, CA 95610

Paperback ISBN: 979-8-218-58922-6
eBook ISBN: 979-8-218-60737-1

Website: www.myimperfectheart.com

Portions of this book were supported with and researched using AI tools, patient and doctor interviews.

Author photo by Ed Goldman.

Special thanks to the founders of Podium, Paul Bloch and Kenneth Miller, for allowing me to work with their chapterization product in beta to craft some of the content from original audio. The product rocked. https://podium.page

Praise for the Podcast: "Imperfect Heart"

It's nice to have the support of someone so positive and to hear all the positive stories you produce. It helps more than you know. You're a hero. You've made such a difference to so many. Myself included.
K.S. - California

I'm crying. You are a rock star. Thank you.
S.M. - California

This is amazing, congratulations on such a great podcast.
Dr. Mark Francis Berry
Stanford University Medical Center

This is giving hope and education to so many. It is a giant leap forward for our myocardial bridge community. Only positive things can come from this. Just imagine how many people would continue to suffer without your information and stories.
R.D. - Indiana

Made me tear up. It's so thoughtful and wonderful to be connected to so many people in our community because of you. Thank you.
A.P. - California

Thank you for the podcast!!! We have sent it to many others as it makes things so much easier to explain.
L.A. - Oregon

Excellent work Jeff, I hope more people will benefit in the future from definitive solutions.
Professor Theodoros Kofidis
Hygeia Hospital, Greece

I'm a member of the MB Facebook group and I thoroughly enjoy all of your podcasts and can't thank you enough for the great information you provide.
J.B. - New Jersey

Jeff, this is great. Thanks for all your hard work. I really appreciate it and think it will have a great impact.
Dr. Husam Balkhy
University of Chicago Medical Center

I just wanted to say that listening to your podcast has given me hope that things could get better, and there may be a way out of this. Keep doing what you're doing and spreading the message.
G.H. - United Kingdom

I am currently trying to get a referral to Cleveland Clinic. If only cardiologists would take a look at your podcast, they would be informed and give hope to patients with this condition.
I.P. – Ohio

Jeff, I couldn't stop smiling as I listened to your perfect rendition of our imperfect hearts. My surgery is scheduled and it's all because of you, the doctors you've interviewed and our friends on FB. Thank you for all you do.
T.R. - Washington

Dedication

This book is dedicated to all of us born with symptomatic myocardial bridges—those grappling with angina, chest pain, and other heart attack-like symptoms that have impacted your quality of life with no understanding or comprehension of how or why.

To those just beginning to navigate the path of diagnosis.

To those who have undergone unroofing surgery and rediscovered the vitality and quality of life that can be restored through proper diagnoses and treatment.

And to the compassionate medical professionals—primary care physicians, cardiologists, and cardiothoracic surgeons—who recognize myocardial bridges as a significant cause of symptoms. Your commitment to understanding, diagnosing, and treating this condition with empathy and precision paves the way for a better future for countless patients.

Patient advocacy, persistence, and the proof of success in treatments are the driving forces that will elevate awareness of myocardial bridges. Together, we can not only improve the lives of those impacted but even save lives as this understanding grows.

Finally, to my wife Theresa, for her support, patience and sacrifices made to allow me to complete this project.

From the very bottom of my imperfect heart, may you experience a return to a rhythm of joy in yours.

Contents

Forward ix
Acknowledgements xiii

1   A Ride Too Far 1
2   Decoding the Enigma: My Unexpected Journey with
    Heart Health 5
3   The Call That Changed It All: Venturing Into the Unknown ... 11
4   The Journey to Diagnosis: Tests, Trials, and Tribulations 15
5   Harnessing the Power of Community and Positivity 21

INTERVIEW: THE DOCTORS 25
- DR. INGELA SCHNITTGER: Tell Us All About It 26
- DR. JEFFREY FOWLER: Go Ahead, Provoke Me 47
- DR. MARK FRANCIS BERRY: Permission to Enter 68
- DR. JACK BOYD: Let's Cross That Bridge Together 92
- DR. HUSAM BALKHY: Bring in the Bots 104

INTERVIEW: THE PATIENTS 119
- DR. LINDA CUNNINGHAM: They Didn't Teach
  This In Med School 120
- JEREMY HESTER: Nursing Myself To Death 131
- SARAH MILLER & VERONICA THAXTON:
  When Too Much Becomes Too Much 150
- JED BAKER: A Bridge Too Far 180
- EMILY TEDORE: A Ho Ho Holiday Like No Other 202

- RAISUL ISLAM: A Father's Travel From Bangladesh
  To California 219
- KELLY PORTILLO: The Intersection of Fact and Faith 232

6 What Would You Find If You Spoke With A Genius? 249
7 Back To That Death Ride: Pedaling the Peaks and
Defying the Odds 277
8 Emergence from the Abyss: The Dream 283
9 Reminders: Oh Yes, Don't Let Me Forget, The Reminders 289
10 25 Myths and Misconceptions of Myocardial Bridges 317

Glossary of Terms Related to Myocardial Bridges 327
Photo Pages 336
Medical Disclaimer and Release of Liability 341
About the Author 343
Life Unfolds For Us 345

Forward

Myocardial bridges (MBs) have long captured the attention of cardiologists and researchers for their complex interplay between and among anatomy, physiology, and clinical presentation.

First described centuries ago, these unique congenital anomalies—characterized by the tunneling of coronary arteries within the myocardial tissue—have evolved from being considered mere anatomical curiosities to becoming critical factors influencing coronary artery disease, ischemia, and arrhythmias. Yet, despite significant advancements in medical imaging and therapeutic approaches, myocardial bridges remain enigmatic, underscoring the need for a comprehensive exploration of their multifaceted nature, their frequency of occurrence globally, their seemingly random production of symptoms and both standardization of diagnostic protocol as well as surgical repair.

With this book, I hope to bridge the gap between basic scientific knowledge and clinical practice by presenting detailed conversations and holistic examination of myocardial bridges. You'll find discussions of pathophysiological mechanisms, as well as potential implications for patient care. With contributions from leading experts in cardiology, cardiac surgery, and patient experience the content reflects a multidisciplinary approach that highlights the nuances of diagnosing, managing, and treating MB-related conditions.

One of the fundamental goals of this book is to both support those suffering from a myocardial bridge and to equip clinicians, researchers and the medical community with a thorough understanding of myocardial bridges, the fact that they are real, do cause symptoms and may be the cause of many sudden cardiac deaths.

By dissecting current controversies and addressing knowledge gaps, I hope to inspire new avenues of research and innovation and to provide structure and hope for those with the condition who are looking for solutions—to their deteriorating quality of life, the uncertainty of their symptoms and the constant fear of not knowing whether this condition is going to be their cause of death.

You'll also find case studies and discussions of state-of-the-art interventions, ranging from pharmacological therapies to advanced robotic surgical techniques. These elements provide a practical framework for integrating evidence-based insights into everyday clinical decision-making.

Included in proof of corrective procedures and their successful outcomes are actual patient stories derived from the podcast of the same name as the book, Imperfect Heart, Stories of Myocardial Bridges.

As the field of cardiovascular medicine advances, it's crucial to continually reassess and expand our understanding of myocardial bridges. By doing so, we can move closer to the ultimate goal of personalized, patient-centered care that optimally addresses the complexities of each individual's cardiac anatomy and physiology, better identify the potential for symptoms of those diagnosed with a myocardial bridge and save lives in the process.

With more than 700,000 deaths from heart disease each year and the understanding that 25% (or greater!) of the population is born with a myocardial bridge, doesn't it make sense that there are likely more deaths due to the consequences of a myocardial bridge than the "estimated" 1% that's used in medical discussion?

That's the myth I hope this book begins to bust. That's the optimism I expect to give those desperately trying to get an accurate diagnosis of the symptoms that are currently or have been previously dismissed. That's the motivation I hope to provide the medical community to dig deeper, do more research and recognize that a patient presenting with symptoms that look like a heart attack but have no apparent cause, may have a myocardial bridge. Take them seriously before simply dismissing them.

I extend my deepest gratitude to the contributors whose expertise and dedication, experience and outcomes, have made this book possible. To the readers, I expect this work to serve as a valuable resource that not only enhances your knowledge, sparks curiosity and further inquiry into this cardiac condition, and provides hope for individuals on their quest for an answer, a solution, to what it is that is causing their symptoms, their angina, shortness of breath, radiating pain in the arm, neck or jaw.

Let's recognize each person's story with the assumption it is possibly cardiac-related when all other tests fail. And finally, above all, let's determine, demonstrate and resolve that myocardial bridges can be treated—giving hope to those struggling with the disease and resulting in quality of lives improved and saved.

Jeff Holden
Fair Oaks, California
2025

Acknowledgements

First and foremost, I am profoundly grateful to my wife, Theresa. Without her, much of what has happened may have taken a different course. Babe, I love you. Thank you for your support pre-and post-surgery and for understanding what this process has done for me as we continue this journey together. To say you were encouraging would be a gross understatement. None of it looks the same without you.

To our kids, Derrick, Max and Rose, I appreciate you guys and your concern for my well-being. Bennet and Paige, I now have a good chance I'll see my granddaughters, Isla and Laine, graduate from high school. Raise a couple of cardiac doctors for us all.

A special thank you goes to my Ed-itorial confidant, Ed Goldman, whose attention to detail, creative consult and input pushed me to think differently about what I wanted to accomplish. Your guidance throughout this process has been invaluable.

I also wish to express my gratitude to the doctors who have given and continue to provide so much information on their best practices, especially Dr. Rishi Menon whose sincere interest in determining a cause for my vasospasms led me to his creative approach to get me to Stanford; and Dr. Jack Boyd of Stanford for his confidence the procedure would yield a result that put me back where I was prior to symptoms presenting themselves. I'm beyond thrilled you were correct. Not everyone is so fortunate.

To the patients and their families who have shared their experiences and allowed us to learn from their journeys, your stories have added depth and humanity to this exploration of myocardial bridges and you have not only shown but are also leading the way for others who are following with their own journeys and procedures. This book represents the inspiration many others need to see.

Finally, to my friends and colleagues, I'm grateful for you all. Special recognition needs to go to my podcast producer, Sawyer Milam, who has been with me every step of the way and knows as much as anyone now about myocardial bridges. You can be certain some of what he's experienced was not in the job description!

To you, the reader, thank you for your belief in the importance of this work. It is my hope that this book and the supporting podcast, website and other content serve as a meaningful contribution to the medical community. I hope that they inspire continued progress in understanding and treating myocardial bridges as well as providing hope and positivity to the tens of thousands suffering from the condition around the world.

For giving me a second chance and the blessing of renewed life, a re-birth day, thank you God. My faith has never been stronger.

Could We Have a Word?

You've probably heard this throughout your life: An accurate diagnosis still isn't a cure.

But it's a start.

This is a book about medical and personal discovery. It's my story but also the stories of many patients who came forward to tell their own sagas on my podcast, "Imperfect Heart." This book includes anecdotes and data about the unique birth defect we've shared. Most importantly, it features interviews with physicians on the front line of treating and healing.

You may be experiencing angina, or chest pain, even heart attack-like symptoms that could be caused by this defect and just haven't been properly diagnosed; however, you don't need to have suffered from the malady described here. You may be or have been a caretaker and / or a loved one of someone who has. Or you may be someone with a restless, and healthy curiosity about new frontiers in medical science and eternal human condition.

We begin...

CHAPTER ONE

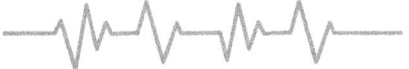

A Ride Too Far

In late July 2021, I was arguably in the best condition of my adult life, having trained all summer for a grueling cycling event at the end of the month. I was fired up. I felt great and I couldn't wait to ride.

When the day came, unfortunately, or possibly fortunately, as you'll learn, the ride had to be canceled due to an explosive fire that erupted the day before.

That fire may have saved my life. The next few weeks began to unfold as a story that would certainly change my life forever.

With the cancellation of the Death Ride, yes, that's what it's called, in July of 2021 I figured I was going to keep up my fitness level and ride out more frequently with my cycling group and get a little more competitive. When you're 65 years old every opportunity to beat somebody with fewer gray hairs is a point of pride and, sure, bravado.

But something happened on my next training ride, and it happened several more times before I was smart enough to get to the doctor to check it out.

I'm sure most of us don't want to admit something might be wrong and we figure we'll just work through whatever it is until we can't. I'm pretty sure we call that denial.

I had developed a searing pain in the center of my chest that would occur right when I was starting out for a ride. Initially, it was just an annoyance. It was only a couple of minutes long and it didn't reflect on any of my monitors as anything odd. It was just very, very uncomfortable. Surely nothing serious. But with each successive ride, that pain lasted longer and it seemed more severe.

Naturally, I would ride through it. If I didn't know any better, I would think it was something to do with my heart but I'm in such good shape it couldn't be.

Finally, it occurred to me that this was something I needed to get looked at. You really shouldn't be anticipating how long you're going to have to deal with it until you can get in with the group again, I thought.

On Monday, August 23rd, I went to my primary care physician and I had some x-rays done and had an EKG taken, set an appointment with the cardiologist for Friday, the 27th.

I never kept that meeting on Friday because I had a myocardial infarction. A heart attack. There. I said it. A heart attack on Thursday morning.

That incident set off a series of tests, return hospital visits, specialists, various drug therapies, cardiac rehab, and finally several other life-threatening heart issues that not only made no sense, but were also getting inaccurately diagnosed with the idea that a remedy was just a few tests away. Sound familiar to you? I would eventually get diagnosed with severe endothelial dysfunction, severe vasospasms, a myocardial bridge and a blockage in the left anterior descending or (LAD) artery, as the culprits of my symptoms.

What transpired and where I am today is a story this book tells. It also tells stories from the experience of cardiologists. It tells stories of medical professionals familiar with myocardial bridges talking about the symptoms these bridges can create.

I'll include stories from other professionals familiar with those suffering from myocardial bridges and the treatments they've endured with successful outcomes, not only physically, but mentally as well.

I'll present stories from patients and caregivers, real stories of the challenges and symptoms a myocardial bridge diagnosis creates. This book is not meant to discourage, it's to encourage. My intent in sharing these experiences is to give everyone with this condition hope. Genuine hope. Knowing that there are others like you that have similar situations. Hope. Knowing others who have benefited from treatment and are sharing their journey. Hope. Knowing that more and more physicians are recognizing myocardial bridge symptoms as something more than just stress or anxiety.

Is it possible that many sudden cardiac deaths could have been or are still being caused by undiagnosed myocardial bridges? More and more is known each and every day. More and more surgeons are practicing the process of unraveling the mystery of a myocardial bridge. More and more of us, those with bridges, are being relieved of some, if not all of our symptoms of the bridge.

Catching the culprit of heart conditions early is critical. I look forward to helping get these stories told and changing, maybe even saving, lives in the process.

In Chapter 2, I speak with my first cardiologist in the process of diagnosis, Dr. Rishi Menon. We had thought what I had was going to be a typical blockage inside a coronary artery causing an interruption in blood supply to the heart muscle, leading to heart muscle damage that showed up on a blood test. We thought we were going to do the standard process or procedure. We did the standard tests, angiogram and cardiac cath. What we were anticipating was that we were talking about some obvious or demonstrable narrowing of the coronary artery. Typically, that's within the acute setting of blood clot or plaque blockage, but we didn't see any of that. I had very normal looking coronaries on this test. There was some slight variation on the angiogram, but nothing that we thought would explain my symptoms at that time.

My journey was now begun.

CHAPTER TWO

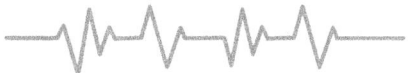

Decoding the Enigma: My Unexpected Journey with Heart Health

THERE I WAS, LYING IN A HOSPITAL BED, MY BODY A LIVING MYSTERY that baffled even the medical professionals around me.

A typical day had taken an unexpected turn when I found myself "presenting" with abnormal heart symptoms. My heart was singing a strange tune, a medley of triplet beats of ventricular tachycardia, alarming enough to land me in the hospital. My friend, Dr. Menon, was summoned, and while he wasn't on call that day, he happened to be in the hospital.

Dr. Menon's arrival felt like, if you'll excuse the expression, a stroke of luck. He didn't expect to see me, an active and ostensibly healthy individual, in such a state. To him, I didn't fit the mold of a typical cardiac patient. My situation was indeed an enigma. Initial tests indicated potential damage to my heart muscle cells, revealed through an abnormal outcome of a blood test indicating a high level of troponin, a protein the leaks into the bloodstream when the cells of the heart become damaged as a result of a heart attack. The cause of this damage, however, was yet to be discovered.

Like detectives on a high-stakes case, we started collecting clues of my heart condition. The first suspicion was an almost generic heart attack—a sudden blockage of a coronary artery with a blood clot, a fairly common occurrence even in younger individuals. We conducted an angiogram, expecting to find this clot or a significant narrowing of the coronary. To our surprise, the results showed normal-looking coronaries, throwing our initial theory out the window.

With the traditional suspects ruled out, we considered alternative theories. One possibility was myocarditis, where the heart muscle is irritated or inflamed, causing damage not due to interrupted blood supply but because of a direct attack on the muscle itself. Armed with this hypothesis, we started some medications, hoping they would alleviate my symptoms.

Yet, as days passed, the medications seemed to be firing blanks. No matter the alterations in blood pressure medications, beta blockers or calcium channel blockers, my heart refused to relent. As I explained my symptoms to Dr. Menon, I could see the bewilderment in his eyes. He encouraged me to articulate my condition as clearly as possible, emphasizing the importance of patient advocacy in diagnostic journeys like mine. This articulate description, he explained, would aid him in discovering if the root of my problems extended beyond stress, diet, or exercise.

The journey towards understanding my peculiar heart condition was just beginning. Every heartbeat echoed with unanswered questions, every test result added a new layer of complexity. With Dr. Menon by my side, I was ready to face whatever lay ahead, even if it meant deciphering the most cryptic codes of my heart.

My heart had always been my ally, a tireless engine powering me through strenuous cycling trails and endurance races. However, that fateful year in 2021, something shifted. My heart, my trusted comrade, began to send out distress signals that I couldn't decipher. It was a curious and unsettling development, akin to hearing a familiar song play out of tune.

In the beginning, the anomaly was subtle. I would pedal on, dismissing the discomfort as an anomaly, a glitch in an otherwise well-oiled machine. After all, I was in my best shape, training for a grueling ride ironically named the "Death Ride." Yet, with each passing day, the subtle whispers of my body became impossible to ignore. A discomfort, a hitch in my heart's rhythm would creep up post-exercise, and it began to define my daily life.

Dr. Menon was the sounding board for my fears and frustrations. He listened attentively as I articulated my symptoms, the exertional limitations that seemed at odds with my physical fitness. As a seasoned cardiologist, he knew the importance of listening to the patient's narrative. Every detail, every nuance of the symptoms, held clues to the mystery that was my heart condition.

Dr. Menon reminded me that in cardiology, much like detective work, you don't begin by looking for zebras in a field of horses. You start with the common suspects, in this case, coronary disease. Yet, my story was veering off the beaten path, prompting us to consider the zebras, the less common culprits of heart ailments.

While we were navigating this complex terrain, Dr. Menon stressed the importance of communication, of, as mentioned earlier, articulating my experiences by writing them down like a narrative, to help both of us better understand my condition. Reflecting on my symptoms, he suggested, could provide valuable insights for further investigation.

I started to journal my experiences. I wrote about my workouts, how they started off abnormally with discomfort, then seemed to settle down as the workout continued. I noted the intensity of the pain, its frequency, and how my heart would stubbornly refuse to cooperate despite the medications.

As we trudged along our journey of discovery, Dr. Menon proposed we try cardiac rehab. It was like treading on a tightrope, with safety measures in place. We would monitor my heart's rhythm as an outpatient, watching closely for any abnormalities. We hoped this would shed some light on my heart's erratic behavior.

I remember my initial sessions at cardiac rehab. The exercises were basic, almost mundane, but I had to start somewhere. Despite the simplicity, my heart would occasionally throw a tantrum by signaling a triplet of premature ventricular contractions or PVC's, sending the medical team into a frenzy. But with each session, each tiny victory or setback, we were getting closer to understanding the cryptic codes of my heart.

The journey was far from over, the mystery far from solved. As I continued to listen to my body's story, penning down its chapters, I was hopeful—hopeful that Dr. Menon and I would finally decipher the enigma that was my heart.

The mystery deepened with a new clue in the form of an irregular heart rhythm. As Dr. Menon explained, it was a "triplet", a peculiar rhythm during which I would have premature ventricular contractions every third beat, like an unexpected hiccup in the otherwise steady cadence of my heart. This anomaly wasn't inherently dangerous occasionally, but given my ongoing discomfort, it was a sign of an underlying issue that we hadn't yet pinpointed.

In my eager anticipation, each cardiac rehab session was tinged with hope that the irregularity would manifest while I was wired up to the monitors, allowing us to unlock the mystery of my condition. Despite my optimism, the rogue rhythm remained elusive during the sessions, revealing itself only in the solitude of my daily life.

I vividly recall a particular day at rehab. The session went smoothly, my heart behaved, and I left feeling optimistic, maybe even relieved. But as I climbed the stairs to the rooftop garage where I'd parked, a familiar sensation crept up on me. The discomfort, the unyielding hitch in my heart rhythm, resurfaced, lingering for an agonizing four minutes. It was an intense episode. The elusive rhythm continued to taunt us, hiding just beyond our grasp. What it did do however, was record and send information to the control center monitoring my heart through a "Holter" monitor which is a small device you wear for a predetermined amount of time that captures your heart's rhythm. Many of you will become familiar with this device on your quest for a solution to your symptoms.

That same day as I arrived at my office, I received a call from Dr. Menon. The monitor had picked up a rhythm called ventricular tachycardia—an alarming, prolonged sequence of abnormal beats or PVC's (premature ventricular contractions) that indicated a severely unhappy heart muscle. This wasn't a benign anomaly anymore, it was a loud and clear signal that something was indeed wrong, potentially linked to a coronary issue or maligned electrical signals controlling my heart's rhythm. The game had changed. Sustained PVC's could lead to ventricular fibrillation where the heart beats so fast, no blood is passed through it, you could then pass out and if not corrected, die.

So, with this revelation, our path took a new turn. It was no longer just about deciphering an irregular rhythm or managing an odd discomfort. I was facing the harsh reality of a potentially life-threatening heart condition. Despite mounting concern, there was a strange sense of relief. We finally had tangible evidence, a solid lead in the enigma of my imperfect heart.

CHAPTER THREE

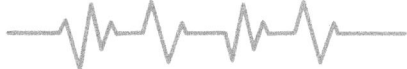

The Call That Changed It All: Venturing Into the Unknown

THE DAY I RECEIVED THAT CALL FROM DR. MENON, MY WORLD tilted on its axis. Sitting at my desk, engrossed in work, I had no idea that the conversation about to unfold would steer my life into an entirely new direction. The seriousness in Dr. Menon's voice struck me, signaling that my heart condition was far more critical than I had anticipated.

Following his instructions, I rushed to the hospital for a cardiac MRI (Magnetic Resonance Imaging), only to find myself caught in an absurd sequence of events. Lying in the MRI machine, a spectacle unfolded around me as the brand-new machine suddenly broke down. The sight of the medical staff scrambling around, coupled with the eerie silence of the malfunctioning machine, was a jarring experience, to say the least.

To complicate matters further, the contrast dye had already been injected for the MRI which necessitated a quick transition to another machine before the dye lost its efficacy. Despite the discomfort and anxiety, we managed to get the test done, hoping it would bring us closer to a definitive diagnosis.

Dr. Menon and his team then dove into a meticulous review of the various tests—the angiogram, CT scans, echocardiogram, and finally, the cardiac MRI. Despite their efforts, a concrete diagnosis eluded us. The mystery deepened when a ventricular tachycardia specialist, an electrophysiologist, agreed that my condition was atypical after reviewing series upon series of EKG results. The puzzle pieces just weren't fitting together.

As we kept tugging at the threads of my heart's peculiarities, a new possibility emerged—a myocardial bridge. It was suggested that my coronary artery, instead of arching over my heart muscle, was tunneling through it. At first, this was casually dismissed as an irrelevant anomaly, a benign condition. The electrophysiologist thought at first these vasospasms were something electrical but quickly suggested more testing was necessary. The more I thought about it, the more I wondered—was this innocuous "birth defect" somehow connected to my symptoms? Was my heart muscle inadvertently squeezing my artery with each beat, disrupting the blood flow? The internet had become my new best friend as I was constantly searching for definitive answers to this condition, a myocardial bridge.

These questions led us down a new path, opening a whole new realm of possibilities. The hunt for answers became more intense and we began exploring the potential of my visiting a more advanced center with specialized expertise in coronary anomalies and vasospasms.

The uncertainty was overwhelming, but I held onto hope. I felt (and hoped) we were making progress, that every question was bringing us one step closer to understanding my imperfect heart. This was not just a medical journey anymore; it was a quest for answers, a pursuit of truth, a story of resilience in the face of the unknown.

THE CALL THAT CHANGED IT ALL

When faced with an unsolved medical puzzle, the world of medicine offers a multitude of tests and procedures to tease out the truth. Dr. Menon suggested a provocative test—a medical procedure designed to elicit or simulate symptoms for diagnosis. In my case, the test aimed to induce spasms in my coronary artery to determine if that was causing my heart issues.

A provocative test is not your average medical exam. It's an advanced procedure that requires a specialist's deft touch and keen eye for nuances. If done right, the test can help diagnose conditions that might otherwise remain hidden, providing critical information for treatment planning. The specialists conducting the test would use specific agents known to cause arterial spasms, aiming to trigger a response in my reactive arteries.

The intriguing aspect of my case was that I was resistant to anti-spasm agents—an unexpected twist that deepened the medical mystery. If the spasms were the root cause of my symptoms, the anti-spasm agents should have provided some relief, but they didn't. This resistance pointed to something more complex, prompting us to seek further specialist advice.

With this decision, the pursuit of a diagnosis became a collaborative effort. Along with Dr. Menon, other cardiologists, and a ventricular tachycardia specialist, we put our heads together, weighing different possibilities. The consensus was clear—my condition was atypical and required further investigation.

As I found myself at the center of this medical conundrum, the possibility of receiving an implanted defibrillator was brought up. This device could potentially save my life if my heart went into ventricular tachycardia, but the thought of living with it felt daunting. It seemed like a last resort, a safety net for when all else fails. But were we really there yet? Was there no other way to understand and manage my condition? I wanted a solution to the problem, not a mask to the symptom and was emphatic, that until we knew the root cause, we would work with only temporary solutions.

Fortunately, I have an incredible wife who was also steadfast in her support and agreement. It was the evening of the same day that the electrophysiologist came into the hospital room to give me his suggestion that the defibrillator was likely my best option, that he returned to explain the various types of defibrillators. That evening was one of the lowest points in the journey as he had no real answers, no optimism and a very somber presentation. It wasn't until the next morning that several cardiologists returned after conversations with Dr. Menon and agreed, there may be another step necessary. My spirits were lifted.

In pursuit of answers, I dove headfirst into researching myocardial bridges - the peculiar anomaly found in my heart. Every new piece of information continued to lead me further down this path of discovery. Meanwhile, the medical team considered different hospitals known for their expertise in coronary anomalies and vasospasms—Cleveland Clinic, Mayo Clinic, and Stanford Medical Center. Given my location in Sacramento, California, Stanford, about two hours away, was my obvious first choice. Stanford also happened to have a research team dedicated to myocardial bridges, which you learn more about in the chapters ahead.

However, before any further tests could be conducted, there was one more hurdle to cross—the life vest. This external defibrillator was a temporary solution to keep me safe from sudden cardiac arrest. Despite its life-saving potential, it was cumbersome and uncomfortable. Yet, it was a necessary step in my journey. It was my "best friend" for months and I hated every minute of it as it was a constant reminder that something was terribly wrong with me.

As I navigated through these uncharted waters, I learned to trust the process. I realized that while staying alive was the priority, the quality of life mattered too. It was this pursuit of a better life that kept me and the medical team striving for answers, refusing to settle for the easy way out. Our shared commitment was the beam that lit our path, leading us forward, one cautious step at a time.

CHAPTER FOUR

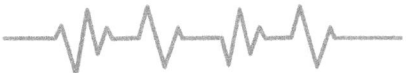

The Journey to Diagnosis: Tests, Trials, and Tribulations

EMBARKING ON THIS MEDICAL ODYSSEY, I KNEW THAT EVERY STEP held the promise of new discoveries. The road was uncertain, peppered with twists and turns. My body's resistance to anti-spasm agents was baffling, only deepening the medical mystery. In collaboration with a team of cardiologists and a ventricular tachycardia specialist, we journeyed through the unknown, hunting for answers.

As we continued our quest, my medical team and I made several critical decisions. The first was to try the life vest—a temporary, external defibrillator. Wearing it felt like donning a bulletproof jacket, complete with a nine-pound battery pack. It was an encumbrance, but a necessary one. Its purpose? To protect me from sudden cardiac arrest while we sought more answers.

Next, we set our sights on Stanford Medical Center. Known for its expertise in coronary anomalies and vasospasms, this was the perfect place to further our investigation. After a few phone calls and paperwork, we got the green light. I found myself admitted to Stanford, poised for provocative testing under the capable hands of Dr. Jennifer Tremmel.

During this testing phase, I experienced spasms and went into ventricular tachycardia while undergoing an echocardiogram. Despite the fleeting hope that we might catch the anomaly in action, the echo didn't reveal much. But it was a critical moment—it provided the first tangible evidence of my condition in a clinical setting. It also scared the hell out the poor young woman doing the echo as the nurse that was monitoring me was watching the EKG showing the VT (ventricular tachycardia), the alarms are sounding and I grabbed her hand and said keep going. Just keep doing your thing. We need to see what shows up. I finally had confirmation that was in a clinical setting for all to see and review. I knew I was in good hands.

Reflecting on this journey, I realized the immense power of patient advocacy. You need to be your own best advocate, vocalizing your experiences and persistently seeking answers. If you can't communicate your symptoms and experiences effectively, it becomes nearly impossible for anyone to help you. It was this advocacy, coupled with the dedication of my medical team, and a wife that was a pit bull on the process, that led us to the truth.

As Dr. Menon and I dug into the details of my case, we realized the importance of seeking multiple perspectives. There were instances when we hit dead ends, when the data didn't add up, when the tests didn't show what we expected. But we never gave up. We continued to ask questions, seek expert opinions, and remain open to new possibilities.

The information we received from Dr. Tremmel as a result of the provocative testing was game-changing. My spasms were severe, my endothelial dysfunction was severe (the condition that causes the artery to spasm) disrupting a significant amount of blood flow. At its worst, 98% reduction in flow rate! This is where the ischemia was coming from. My LAD had significant enough blockage at the point of entry to the heart that it also necessitated a coronary artery bypass graft or CABG procedure. These findings made everything fall into place—it explained why I developed ventricular tachycardia and why the anti-spasm medications weren't working. This was the cause of the constant pain and the trigger that could have led to my untimely death. The pieces of the puzzle finally began to fit together.

Through it all, I was reminded of the strength of shared experiences. It was a journey marked by uncertainty and anxiety, but it was also a journey of discovery and hope. It reinforced the notion that in the face of a medical mystery, persistence, advocacy, and collaboration are the keys to unlocking the answers.

In the wake of my diagnosis, I found myself standing on a precipice, staring into a sea of uncertainty. There was a semblance of relief, a faint flicker of understanding. But what lay ahead was still shrouded in shadows. The spasms were causing my pain, yet the myocardial bridge remained a question mark. At this juncture, I can't help but express my deep gratitude to Dr. Menon. His wisdom and guidance illuminated my path, providing clarity amidst the confusion.

As I began to find a path through this intricate maze of health and healing, I discovered a dimension often overlooked in the clinical realm—the spiritual. For many, including myself, spirituality is an integral part of the healing journey. It's a sanctuary, a wellspring of strength when the physical and emotional toll becomes overwhelming. It offers solace and serenity, irrespective of individual religious beliefs.

In addition to spiritual support, the power of shared experiences can't be overstated. After revealing my condition to a friend, a cardiac nurse, she admitted complete unfamiliarity with it. She'd never heard of my condition; this strange thing called a myocardial bridge. A few days later, she returned with news that made my heart skip a beat (not literally, of course, well…maybe it did!). Another cardiac nurse, a friend of hers, had a friend who had the same condition. The prospect of connecting with someone who'd been through the same storm brought a rush of hope, an overwhelming sense of optimism.

Speaking with this marathon runner, who'd undergone the same unroofing procedure I was to be considering, was an enlightening experience. Our conversation, stretching over two hours, was a profound testament to the bond forged by shared experiences. She painted a picture of optimism and resilience, instilling in me a belief that there was light at the end of this tunnel. It wasn't just the conversation itself, but the ripple effects it created, steering me towards the next steps in my journey. You'll read of our conversation later in the book.

It's my fervent hope that this book will bring a similar ray of hope to those wrestling with medical mysteries. Advocacy, meticulous documentation, relentless questioning, and the unyielding pursuit of answers can pave the way towards diagnosis and healing.

Dr. Menon echoed this sentiment, underscoring the significance of shared experiences. No one should navigate these challenging paths alone. Finding communities of people grappling with similar conditions can bring practical advice, the comforting knowledge of not being alone, and a spiritual connection that soothes the soul.

And this isn't confined to physical spaces. I found solace in a private Myocardial Bridge Support Group on Facebook (yes, it really exists): global community where shared concerns and experiences spanned across geographical boundaries. Here, you were encouraged to voice your fears and concerns without judgment, drawing strength from a supportive network.

In retrospect, my gratitude for Dr. Menon knows no bounds. I'm deeply appreciative of his unwavering support and guidance, his tireless efforts in saving lives, and for joining me on this life-altering journey. Despite the unusual circumstances that led to our friendship, I'm immensely grateful for the bond we've forged and the journey we continue to traverse together.

CHAPTER FIVE

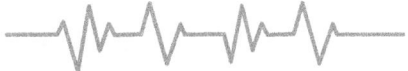

Harnessing the Power of Community and Positivity

As I write this, sharing my journey with you, I am filled with an overwhelming sense of gratitude and hope. The purpose of these shared experiences and conversations, is to not only inform but also to uplift. I want you to understand that no matter the depth of your struggles, you are never alone.

There are communities of individuals, just like you, grappling with the same uncertainties and fears. They are there, waiting to welcome you, to share their stories and lend a comforting ear. I found solace in the private Myocardial Bridge Support Group on Facebook, in that one person at the time that I was able to speak with in person and a network of individuals bound by shared experiences. This platform transcends geographical boundaries, uniting hearts from across the globe. If you, too, are battling with a myocardial bridge diagnosis, I strongly urge you to seek out this community and now, you also have the benefit of the podcast I created for us, those with myocardial bridges. The "Imperfect Heart" community. Global as well, these are real conversations with real people and real doctors helping each and every one of us. Available on most podcast apps and YouTube, the podcast is the living extension of the digital conversations taking place on Facebook. It's the natural compliment. The website, www.myimperfectheart.com, is a continuous work in progress and will house additional information to help you along on your journey.

If you are looking for more information, or if you wish to connect with me directly, you can find my information on the website. Here, I aim to provide a resource that guides you through your journey, offering hope and support along the way.

The process towards healing is often paved with challenges, but it's important to remember the power of positivity. Embrace each day with a heart full of gratitude. Despite the difficulties, try to focus on the small victories, the sparks of light that pierce through the dark clouds of uncertainty.

The conversations that follow, these shared experiences, are meant to shed light on the labyrinth of cardiac care, to offer you a sense of direction when everything else seems blurry. But remember, while I share my journey and insights with you, these are solely my views and those of the interviewees. They are not intended to replace professional care or advice. Always consult with a healthcare professional for medical advice and treatment. Nothing in these chapters is meant to be anything more than information or even a bit of entertainment. We have to laugh at some of what takes place or we'll lose our minds. I also want to give you permission to feel. Be aware of your feelings, share them, cry when you need to, want to. Scream! Louder! You're going to want to do a fair amount of that to be sure. And talk. Don't hold it all in. There's no need. There are plenty of people willing to listen. Find humor wherever you can. Laughter truly is the best medicine. I'll just caution you here that if you have a sternotomy as your procedure for unroofing, that laughter is going to hurt early on but it's so worth it. Be your authentic self in the process as you're going to be stripped down to the essence of your life. There's no need for a mask here. That's too much work. Be you. It's OK to experience every emotion possible. It will lighten your load to recovery. I promise. It was difficult for me and I'm told I'm different as a result. I know it. For others to see it as well is confirmation. I mean that for the better.

I am humbly inviting you to join me on this journey. If you find value in these conversations, please do share them with those close to you. You never know whose life you might touch, whose path you might illuminate. Don't forget to subscribe to the podcast to stay updated on our journeys together. Your engagement and support serve as reminders that in our shared struggles, we find shared strength.

What follows are transcripts of my podcast, "Imperfect Heart," conducted from January, 2023 to December, 2024.

I've edited these for clarity and to minimize redundancy, not for content. I'm profoundly grateful for the permission of all the participants to share their stories and I appreciate the contributions they have all made in telling their stories, doctors and patients alike.

Not everyone who goes through a traumatic, life-altering, highly emotional experience—whether it's losing a loved one, barely escaping death or, as is the case here, successfully crossing the myocardial bridge to safety—is willing to or, often times, even capable of sharing what they felt or learned. This is understandable: Why force yourself to relive the terror, pain or trauma of the event or occurrence?

I think that the answer is this: the medical professionals and patients who agreed to speak with me shared something more significant than an interest in infirmity. They shared a desire to help their fellow human beings.

Let me share these stories.

THE INTERVIEWS

Edited Transcripts From "Imperfect Heart" Podcast Episodes

THE DOCTORS

DR. INGELA SCHNITTGER: Tell Us All About It

(Her personal story of myocardial bridge discovery and her subsequent action.)

Imagine a condition so common that it affects 25 percent or more of the population—yet is so complex that its diagnosis and treatment require an interdisciplinary effort.

This is the world of myocardial bridges, a realm of cardiology that has intrigued and baffled many. Enter Stanford's Dr. Ingela Schnittger.

Dr. Schnittger is a trailblazer in the field with an academic and medical background that spans continents and disciplines. She is a familiar figure to many in the myocardial bridge community, having dedicated her career to understanding this often confused and confusing cardiovascular condition and advocating for patients. Her commitment led to the formation of a dedicated myocardial bridge research team at Stanford University, contributing to the fact that unroofing surgery—a surgical procedure to treat myocardial bridges—is now performed in an increasing number of hospitals worldwide. How her interest in this condition came to be is where I begin the conversation I had with her.

Jeff Holden (Host): You are an icon in the field and provide such hope for so many still working to get a proper diagnosis of their symptoms or working to find a surgeon to perform their unroofing. Welcome to Imperfect Heart. Could you please share what it was that caused you to begin down this path of learning about myocardial bridges?

Dr. Ingela Schnittger (Guest): I was asked to be a medical expert in a legal case in which a young man had exercise-induced chest pain. He had a treadmill test. That was normal. His primary care doctor reassured him but he continued to have exercise-induced chest pain. One day, while he was running on a treadmill in a commercial gym, he had a sudden cardiac arrest. He was resuscitated but turned out to be brain dead. The autopsy showed a myocardial bridge with a plaque upstream from the bridge that had ruptured and formed a clot around it and he had an acute heart attack followed by an arrhythmia that caused the heart to stand still. I was supposed to be the expert on the defendant side. But the plaintiff's attorney who took my deposition knew everything about myocardial bridges and I knew nothing. It was humbling, it was embarrassing and it came to really pique my interest. What is this myocardial bridge and why is it that it wasn't diagnosed? That's what got me started.

JH: It's interesting that the legal and medical fields come together, as they do so often and in this case, for the greater good. What then led you to the research at Stanford and formalizing this into a myocardial bridge team?

Dr. Ingela Schnittger: Well, I'm a specialist in cardiac ultrasound, also called echocardiography, and so I interpret echocardiograms and have done so for 40 years. One day I'm sitting in the lab and I'm reviewing a file of a 35-year-old man who came to the lab for chest pain and had an exercise echocardiogram, and as I was looking at the pictures, I was struck by an abnormal motion of one of the walls of the heart. He reminded me of my legal case, so I asked myself could this be a pattern of motion in a person with a myocardial bridge? When it turned out that he soon thereafter *did* have an invasive angiogram that *did* show a myocardial bridge, this then highlighted my interest in studying this condition. I wanted to do invasive angiograms for patients that had this pattern and of course I had to team up with another specialist, specifically Dr. Jennifer Tremmel, an invasive cardiologist, and a team of fellows helped us get started on investigating the bridges in the cath lab, and then we realized we needed intravascular ultrasound.

We engaged our very superb intravascular ultrasound laboratory that eventually led to involving a cardiac surgeon. That's how we formed the team, and because the myocardial bridges are much more complicated than meets the eye, you need input from different specialties. I should also say that we were working with the radiologist who did the CT scans, they learned from us and we learned from them what constitutes a significant myocardial bridge. That's how we came to form the whole team. I think it's important to have this team approach because there are aspects of a bridge that even a cardiologist isn't going to know all the intricacies in evaluating.

JH: I can't help but think back again to the gentleman on the treadmill whose heart attack started this cause for research and a myocardial bridge, yet, so many times and so frequently, we're told it's benign.

Dr. Ingela Schnittger: Well, it's interesting because, as you probably know, myocardial bridging is very common. Depending on the tool that you use to study the heart, at least 20 to 25% of all people out there will have some degree of myocardial bridging. But there's a wide variability in the severity of the bridging. The length, the depth, how hard the band compresses the vessel, how many side branches are jailed in the tunnel segment, how hard the band presses on the heart. We have also shown it's correlated to plaque buildup. After you form the plaque, that then becomes a problem. There are so many aspects which make it very challenging to sort out what bridge is likely to cause symptoms and what kind of situation should we worry about? The heart attack situation, right? There are several pieces to this. It's not just one-shoe-fits-all.

JH: Dr. Tremmel did my provocative test to identify the symptoms and cause and what was happening. How long ago did you start the team at Stanford? And, at what point did you decide, hey, we can actually do repair as well, we can do the surgery on these things as well as diagnosing and understanding them better?

Dr. Ingela Schnittger: Well, it wasn't quite so simple as to say, okay, we just build a team and then go from there. It was a series of things that developed. We learn with every little project we do. But we had a surgeon involved pretty quickly after we started to diagnose the bridges as significant from a circulatory problem. In the beginning we had a couple of surgeons, but in the last eight years we've had one single surgeon who does all the surgeries. Surgeons want to have some reassurance that the bridge is actually causing a circulatory problem, since bridges are common and many of them do not cause a circulatory problem.

The surgeons, understandably, were tentative in doing open heart surgery. It's not a walk in the park, it's a major surgery and you don't want to harm anybody. "Do no harm" is the number one epic concept we have. The surgeons wanted to have confirmation that there was a circulatory problem and it was challenging to prove a circulatory problem because everything that had been done up to that point was to study circulatory problems in fixed blockages, fixed coronary artery disease, fixed blockages. The bridge is a very dynamic situation. If you study the bridge at rest—a patient on the table in the catnap—sedated, slow heart rate, you may find nothing. We had to move to the concept of studying a bridge under the circumstances that are real life experience, such as exercising, and it could be just walking up to an upstairs apartment, but a situation where you're moving, okay? That was the first obstacle, and as we were able to prove that with a new measurement tool, we got surgery on board.

JH: Why do you think that there's still such a lack of understanding about the symptoms of bridges when now you've got, what, 10, 12 years of history, surgery correction and proper diagnosis? It still seems to be vague in the cardiology community.

Dr. Ingela Schnittger: Yes, I agree with you and I think, first and foremost, as I mentioned, you had to use different tools to prove that there is a circulatory problem. Okay? You have to study the artery during induced stress that we do in the cath lab. Secondly, I think that a majority of the patients that have a significant myocardial bridge do have endothelial dysfunction. What is endothelial dysfunction? Well, the lining of the vessel is made up of special cells called endothelial cells and in order for the blood vessel to stay open all the time, those endothelial cells have to be healthy. They produce nitric oxide, which keeps the vessels open.

When you bang on that vessel every minute, every second, with compression of the heart muscle, you traumatize the endothelial lining and you have a tendency to develop spasms. Why is that important? Because the spasm is random, it occurs when you're at rest, it can wake a person up at night. It comes with emotional stress and physical stress, too.

The problem here is that the patient, the person afflicted by this condition, has chest discomfort, with effort and at rest. If you go to a doctor and say you have chest pain, they're going to say okay, let's see, do you have any risk factors for coronary artery disease. Maybe this is GERD (acid reflux), whatever. Maybe you end up saying, okay, well, it's pretty typical pain from the heart. But when you say you get pain watching a movie or talking to your partner or spouse or kid, then the doctor is going to say, uh-uh, this is not typical. You're probably just a little stressed, you're a little bit, you know, anxious. This is not heart disease. That's the problem. Then people get dismissed. It's the symptomatology—with pain, both with effort and rest, as well as it being a very common condition—challenging to sort out which bridges are causing problems. In order to study that, you have to understand that this is a dynamic situation and you have to apply different diagnostic tools.

JH: I can certainly agree with the "at rest" part, because most of my spasms occurred, initially, when I was at rest. I had my myocardial infarction, which is so hard to say I had a heart attack, but I had that heart attack in the morning waking up in bed.

Dr. Ingela Schnittger: Yes.

JH: Nothing to do with stress or exercise. As a matter of fact, when I exercised it was better.

Dr. Ingela Schnittger: Right.

JH: I never even had the symptoms under heavy exercise.

Dr. Ingela Schnittger: This variability in the symptom, when you go to the doctor with chest pain—doctor of primary care, internal medicine, cardiologist-and you see chest pain, it's incumbent upon the doctor to go through the differential list, right, to tell the patient that it's musculoskeletal. Musculoskeletal pain is painful to touch. When you press on the chest it hurts. Heart pain does not hurt from the surface. If the pain is coming from the heart, you cannot elicit the pain by pushing on the muscle. There are a number of ways you can narrow down the potential differential diagnosis because of chest pain. I mean, every patient who walks through my office door has chest pain of some sort or another. It's a common problem, right? We need to do better in asking questions that might lead you down the road to the question, "Could it be a myocardial bridge?"

JH: Is there one gold standard that identifies the fact that, yes, this is a myocardial bridge with enough severity to cause symptoms?

Dr. Ingela Schnittger: I think that the most reliable non-invasive test is the CT scan. And we have shown that if you do a careful CT scan with controlled heart rate, you want the heart rate to be 60 or less, otherwise you get fuzzy pictures when the heart moves. So, you do a good CT scan and from the CT scan you can measure the length and you can estimate the depth. We have developed a myocardial bridge muscle mass index. It's basically a number and if that number hits a certain threshold, and we have compared that to invasive studies, so then we can say, okay, if your muscle mass index is X, it's a very high likelihood that you have a circulatory problem in your bridge.

I recommend that after you do stress testing, which I can come back to, which could be positive or negative, I would say the next step is a CT scan. Then you have to have a radiologist who's going to read it. I even have radiologists at Stanford who don't always read the bridge because they are so in the mode of thinking it's so common, it's a normal variant, we don't need to bother. I've had to say to my radiology colleagues I only want Dr. X, Y or Z to read them, because if I want to see the scan and if somebody else will receive the scan when the question is chest pain, please pay attention.

JH: It actually is a specific look that they get with the experience of doing more and more and more, obviously, right? Certainly, you've got to be extremely proud of your accomplishments to date and ongoing. What do you think needs to be done to get more of the data that you're coming up with and providing it to cardiologists around the world, so that we can help more people with this?

Dr. Ingela Schnittger: I do think that the condition, the subject, is getting some traction, and I think it's multifactorial. I think we have published a good deal. There are actually more publications from abroad than from American institutions, sadly to say. I think that there is an increasing awareness in the cardiology medicine community, but I also think that your work and Facebook is also helping people to gain more understanding. We get a lot of referrals from across the country and sometimes from abroad.

When I ask the patient, how did you come to Stanford? They would say well, "I struggled for many years. I eventually got the diagnosis that I have a myocardial bridge, but I was told that don't worry, it's not causing your symptoms. Then I go online and I find out that it could be a problem." So sometimes it's the patient who's pushing for more consultation or second opinion. Sometimes it's the cardiologist saying "Oh, I see that you have a myocardial bridge. I don't know if it's causing your symptom, I don't know enough about it, but let's send you to another institution for a second opinion." There are two ways that they come, and I think that is increasing.

In the beginning, most of my patients were local, but now most of my patients are from out of state and they come because they understand they may have a problem, or their doctor, I would say, admits or acknowledges that they may have a problem. I think it's happening. It's still sort of tentative in some people's mind, but I think we're making progress.

JH: I would definitely say you're making progress, and the recognition of Stanford as the leader in the diagnosis and the process of remedy to the extent that it can be remedied, is world-renowned, especially from the Facebook group, our interviews with patients and doctors on the podcast and how people are now recognizing it. I had a gentleman from India email me and ask me, "What do you know about Stanford, what can you tell me?" because he can't find a doctor in India to do the surgery. It's something you should be extremely proud of. So, thank you, thank you, thank you. Keep going.

Dr. Ingela Schnittger: I think we've gone forward slowly and cautiously. I feel very sorry for a surgeon who is just approached by a patient who says I have a myocardial bridge; can you fix it? Because my surgeon, he would not take a patient to surgery unless the team says this is a problem. We have studied this individual. There's a high likelihood that he or she will improve with surgery. We need to make sure there are no other major issues. We do very careful mapping of the bridges to let the surgeon know exactly where the bridge starts, where it ends, how long is it? My surgeon, he even takes out a measurement in the operating room after he has dissected from the bridge and he measures and he says, okay, Ingela, I have 31 millimeters, Is that good enough?

Even I, as a cardiologist, have learned a lot going to the operating room and you would think that if you open up the breastbone and you look at the heart, that it would be absolutely obvious where the bridge is. Uh-uh, no, no, because it can be covered in fat in the pericardium, you need to know exactly the location, how long it is, what your landmarks are. From the CT scan we learn if it goes very deep, if it goes into the right ventricle, we have to go on pump. We decide on pump, off pump, mini thoracotomy, sternotomy, all preoperative evaluation so that the surgery can be done with a complete dissection of the whole bridge. Sometimes there are two bridges. You have to do both. It's safe. We haven't lost anybody. No aneurysms of the heart, strokes or heart attacks, because you're very, very, very careful due to the evaluation before the patient goes to surgery. I feel very, very sorry for the surgeon who's asked to just oh, I have a bridge, can you take care of it? This is not some superficially built surgery. It's major and you as a doctor want to instill the confidence in the person, in the patient, that they'll do well, they'll improve and it's a reasonable approach, right?

JH: That was my second question of my surgeon. The first one was, "How many of these have you done?" And he looks at me with a little smile and he says, "Over the course of the last ten years, more than anybody else in the world". I said, oh, okay. I almost felt like I insulted him. But how would you know? I think the significance of that is, when you hear something like that, you say, wow, more than anybody else in the world? That's got to be a lot. At that point in time it was 200… over 10 years! Relatively speaking, that's a lot. By comparison to other surgeries, not so much. In some of the research I've seen and you've confirmed, it's been estimated that roughly 25% or more of the population could be walking around with a myocardial bridge, and it could even be postulated that the cause of many of these blocked coronary arteries resulting in sudden cardiac arrest could be as a result of a bridge that's unrecognized. Is that fair to say?

Dr. Ingela Schnittger: Yes, it's very interesting. Sudden cardiac arrest is not a disease in itself, it's an event, and it's caused by a ventricular arrhythmia. The heart starts to go very, very fast and almost just fibrillating. It goes so fast that it actually doesn't mechanically pump any blood out of the heart. A cardiac arrest can be caused by a number of different conditions. Myocardial bridge is one of them and then there are two aspects of the bridge. Number one is a plaque that everybody I have studied in the cath lab, has small or medium or large, and it's always in the same position and it's regardless of whether you have any risk factors for plaque. They form plaque because of the turbulence in front of the tunneled segment, in front of the bridge.

You could either, like my legal patient, have plaque, plaque rupture and acute 100% occlusion, a heart attack and an arrhythmia, or you can have repetitive chest pain episodes that show the circulation in the bridge and cause fibrosis, scar and edema, swelling. There are autopsy studies where people have looked at patients or people who died in a cardiac arrest. Some of them, of course, do not have a bridge, but then there's a cohort that has a bridge and in those patients they have found scar tissue and edema in the area subtended by the area that is confined in the bridge; that structure is a trigger for ventricular arrhythmias. You can have an acute heart attack. It shows the circulation 100 percent triggers arrhythmia. You can have a build-up of scar and edema inside the heart wall, the septum. That triggers arrhythmia.

It's tricky because you can look at autopsy studies, you can look at, retrospectively, cohorts of people who died in a cardiac arrest and there are bridges there. But, of course, there are several other conditions. When it comes to the bridges you have to look for them because if the pathologist isn't thinking bridge, he's not going to find the bridge. He's going to look for hypertrophic cardiomyopathy, he's going to look for dilating cardiomyopathy, he's going to look for a valvular heart disease, etc. etc. More common things.

Clearly, there are bridges in that cohort, some of them triggered by an acute heart attack, some of them triggered by just the scar tissue, edema that especially with effort—I mean you hear about football players, basketball players, marathon runners who just drop and if they have a bridge and nothing else, it could be either due to just edema, scar or acute plaque rupture. I have one patient who ran the San Francisco marathon, got chest pain, got to a local hospital. The doctor there knew how to study with the angiogram and he had a plaque rupture, he had a heart attack and he had a bridge and he was saved.

JH: I want to dance and I want to scream and I want to shake people, because what you just said in that description is exactly why I stress sooner better than later, because that plaque is only going to get worse over time the longer you wait. It was 65 years for me, which means I had the ability for that plaque to build and I didn't have any other conditions that would suggest that I have an issue. So that was just a wonderful, wonderful description for anybody to understand how this happens.

Dr. Ingela Schnittger: It's interesting because there is a group in Japan that has actually looked at autopsy studies in patients with bridges and acute heart attacks, and it turns out that the plaque in the bridged patients is more vulnerable to plaque rupture and clot formation than the plaque in the same position in another person who doesn't have a bridge. These plaques are vulnerable to fissure and rupture and adhered clot, and so therefore anybody who has a significant bridge should be considered for baby aspirin also.

JH: Yes, I take it every day now.

Dr. Ingela Schnittger: …and also, of course, continuously reviewing any existing risk factors for plaque buildup. Most often it could be cholesterol, because that could be quiet and then the person doesn't know. Diabetes is a risk factor, but people often know that they have diabetes. We treat the cholesterol, we treat with baby aspirin if a person has symptoms, and also, preferably, some diagnosis of the severity of the bridge.

JH: I had the good fortune of a bypass of my LAD (left anterior descending artery) just to really be safe and get around that obstruction. The occlusion was too severe from the plaque buildup to simply unroof me.

Dr. Ingela Schnittger: You had a bypass as well, but that's tricky. It's tricky because, yes, in your case, your plaque was deemed to be partially occluding the vessel.

JH: Yes. 70% occluded, if I recall correctly.

Dr. Ingela Schnittger: You had two problems. You had a plaque that was partially occluding the vessel and then you had a bridge that was partially occluding. Then it's legit to do bypass and unroofing. Please do not bypass a plaque that has not been proven flow limiting, because if you do that the bypass will close. You were fortunate to have a very, very, very careful evaluation that showed your plaque was significant enough that it encroached on the lumen.

See, what happens with these plaque buildups in the bridges is that the vessel enlarges "eccentric", so the plaque doesn't encroach on the lumen until very, very late. It causes a half-moon area of map which changes the size and the shape of the vessel and that's why it goes unrecognized forever. Those plaques don't show up on a CT scan unless they're calcified. Most of them are not calcified. They only show up on an intravascular ultrasound. They don't show up on a coronary angiogram unless they start to encroach on the lumen. But they can still be there, they can still be potentially dangerous. It's tricky. It's very, very tricky and you should never, ever, ever, bypass a plaque that isn't flow limiting. You were very, very, very carefully evaluated and they found that your plaque was limiting the blood flow to that area.

JH: Could you walk us through what you would suggest as a proper diagnosis and course of action? Once I'm aware that I've got this pain, I know it's not fleeting, it's not emotionally originated, it's something material and I may even have gotten the diagnosis that it is but it hasn't been diagnosed as a bridge. What steps would you suggest for somebody in that situation? The first step, second and then, obviously, conclusion.

Dr. Ingela Schnittger: We assume that a person has been evaluated in such a way that you have excluded other causes of the chest pain. You don't have GERD (acid reflux). You don't have musculoskeletal pain. You don't have pericarditis, and hopefully at some point you get either just a simple angiogram or CT scan that shows you have a bridge. I think if you carry that diagnosis, you don't need more testing to start to treat it medically. All bridges should be treated medically first, that's number one.

That's the first line of treatment. You don't really need to know the intricacies of the severity of the bridge to start treatment. The treatment will be number one, the beta blocker, and that reduces the heart rate and the contractile force. If the person doesn't tolerate the beta blocker, maybe a calcium channel blocker, especially if they have a tendency to spasm. Beta blocker plus, minus the calcium channel blocker, then I would really seriously consider a baby aspirin, unless there's a contraindication for aspirin. Then I would check the cholesterol and make sure that the LDL (low-density lipoprotein, the fat that moves cholesterol throughout the body), the bad guy, is better than upper limits of normal. All the patients would say, okay, my LDL is 129 and the upper limit is 130. That's good, right, doc? And I say uh-uh, not good enough.

If you look at the coronary artery disease literature they would say 70 is the best. I may not be as strict to go down to 70, but certainly less than 100, at least in that range. I would start with that. If the patient feels better, they have chest pain less often, it is shorter lasting, they have no show stoppers. Not like if they go on a hike and have to find minutes to stop because they think they're going to die. No, if you can reduce symptoms with those treatments, then I'm happy and the patient is usually happy.

We may increase the dose of whichever medication we believe to have been reducing symptoms then we see them back in a while. If they can do what they want to do and the quality of life is acceptable, then we stop there.

If they fail to improve the quality of life, then I go on to the cath lab and then I do the invasive studies we have talked about. You have to look for endothelial dysfunction. You have to stress the blood vessel to see what happens when the heart rate goes up if you have a circulatory problem. If they have no other issues with their coronary arteries and they test positive for a significant circulatory problem and they've found medical management is not working, then we start to talk about unroofing surgery. But I am very, very, very careful to point out we cannot guarantee you are going to live longer. That's not been shown. We cannot guarantee you can never have a heart attack. That, too, has not been shown.

The surgery is done for symptom reduction, increased quality of life and the patients that end up having the surgery, they, on the average quality of life, have 25% of what they think it should be before surgery, and after surgery, after six months, they're up to 78, 80% quality of life and most people are content with that.

Some people have 100% improvement, maybe some have 70%, and it depends on whether they also have endothelial dysfunction. Endothelial dysfunction does not go away automatically with surgery. What I see clinically is that it improves with time and, I think, because the vessel is not constantly traumatized but endothelial dysfunction tends to be easier to treat. It's not as intense, it's not as frequent, it's not as severe, and then you can often be very successful with low-dose nitrates after surgery. Nitrates before surgery is a little bit dicey because some people get worse. It's a very, very stepwise approach and if they come to me with just chest pain, we start at the bottom of this journey because, as I said, surgery is major and you want it to be safe, you want to have reasonable confidence that the person is going to improve.

JH: If a particular cardiologist is reticent or reluctant to address the reality of the symptoms from a myocardial bridge and that happens to be my particular doctor—I don't mean mine in this case—but I mean anybody who is in that situation, what steps might you suggest for those patients?

Dr. Ingela Schnittger: Stanford happens to have an online second opinion website and it's now actually called Included Health, you can go online and apply and they will help you collect your medical records. They will organize them and they will choose a physician who can review, record and come up with recommendations. You're allowed five questions and so exists not just for my coronary team. It can be, I have prostate cancer. Should I have radiation or surgery, you know, whatever? So that's one way of going.

I think that if you as a patient have been given this diagnosis and you have ongoing symptoms and you've not been helped with medications, then you can certainly ask your doctor for a referral. And if that particular doctor is not sensitive to your request, you can go to another cardiologist and ask for a referral. I's not just Stanford that looks at this. I know people have gone to Mayo, to Cleveland, to Columbia. At least get a second opinion. They may not, my understanding, do that many surgeries, but they certainly can evaluate. I think that you have to say that they have the knowledge to assess the myocardial bridge.

JH: What does the future look like for both diagnosis and treatment of myocardial bridges? What do you think is starting to happen?

Dr. Ingela Schnittger: As I alluded to, I think that the CT scan is an excellent non-invasive tool to get an idea of who may have a significant bridge. I think there is more work to be done to try to non-invasively look at the hemodynamic consequence of a bridge. One aspect that I think is interesting is something called strain imaging. It's an ultrasound technique, perhaps path imaging, different imaging techniques that can address the potential consequence of the bridge. The CT is great because it gives you an anatomic picture and we have correlated that with invasive studies. But it's also good to have a second tool to look at the consequence of the bridge. I think that there are potential tools that can be researched and studied to see if we can assess that better. I think it would be interesting to look at endothelial dysfunction non-invasively because, say that I have a patient with chest pain and we studied them in the cath lab. They have a lot of endothelial dysfunction and the bridge is pretty minor, then surgery is not a good option. They have severe microvascular dysfunction, which is the small vessel disease, and we test that in the lab. If they have a lot of microvascular dysfunction, that can be seen in people with diabetes, smoking, autoimmune disease, transplant patients. There are other conditions that can limit the blood flow to the heart. If you can study those other conditions in a little bit more detail, non-invasively, that will be great. I don't see anything in the near future that would take surgery off the table. It's interesting because people have thought, oh, we can stent the bridge. Okay, that would be cool. People argue that the stent will keep the vessel open so that when the heart contracts the bridge isn't going to be compressed as much. The problem is there are a lot of potential complications with doing that. You can completely compress the stent. Oh, we can build sturdier stents. But that's not going to solve all the problems, because there's one more problem, one more thing.

We have looked at a large cohort, over 100 patients, with significant myocardial bridges, studied in the cath lab that not only do they have a progression, even when the heart contracts, it squeezes, then when the vessel opens, it doesn't open to the same luminal diameter as it should if there wasn't a bridge there. 87% of that cohort of 115 patients had restrictive vessel diameter, even in the relaxed phase. If you put a stent in, it's going to prevent in the beginning, perhaps the systolic compression, but it's not going to be able to overcome the confinement of the vessel segment inside the bridge when the heart relaxes. So that's the problem. I don't see that. The surgeon of course takes away the band of muscle so that in the relaxing phase the vessel can expand. I don't see anything on the near horizon that is going to take surgery off the table. I would recommend to any institution that wants to get into the bridges to create a team and do a careful preoperative assessment, like we have outlined, and stay with one surgeon if possible. You want one guy or gal to become a super expert, because that improves the safety. I believe you had Dr. Boyd, right?

JH: I did, yes.

Dr. Ingela Schnittger: He's the only surgeon I've referred, because he is now probably the world's most experienced and it takes time to get there. I would say focus your referral to one person who has a chance to gain experience and help that surgeon to carefully evaluate your patient before you go to surgery.

JH: Some of the surgeries are being done robotically when possible, a little bit less invasive, a little bit shorter healing time, which is good to see.

Dr. Ingela Schnittger: Yes, I am aware of robotic surgery being done. I think in very experienced hands, somebody who does robotic surgery routinely, it probably can be done safely. I think you really have to customize it to each person. It's not a surgery approach for all people, because you don't want the bridge to be longer than a certain number or deeper, you don't want it to be deep enough that it goes into the right ventricle because you may need to control bleeding. I mean this. I'm getting pretty granular here.

JH: It is a big topic, and it frequently comes up, because people recognize the significance of the sternotomy. If I can do it without all that pain and all that grief. This is good to discuss.

Dr. Ingela Schnittger: Yes, it's good to discuss. About half of our patients are probably in the need for thoracotomy, which is to go in between the ribs and you don't go through the breastbone. The healing, the recovery is quicker. You may just be able to spread the ribs apart and not cut the rib. So that is ideal for a certain group of patients.

Again, it depends on length and depth and position of the bridge. It's easier if you don't have to go on the cardiopulmonary bypass machine. And why do you have to go on that? Well, again, it depends on the location, length and depth of the bridge. So, yes, I think it's a good potential, but with the understanding that it is for a smaller cohort of patients that it can be done safely and also completely right. We have seen patients referred to us who have had a quote, unquote, bridge surgery and it wasn't complete. They still have symptoms. Then do we have a second surgery? So, yes, I think it's interesting, I think it can be done. Seek out somebody who does it for a living, robotic surgery. Be sure that the surgeon understands the anatomy of the problem.

JH: In your years in the field in echocardiograms and cardiology and your familiarity with myocardial bridges, is there any one thing that you've seen in patients that you would say was most important in their process of leading up to a successful recovery from the surgery? You might say health, you might say faith, you might say their relationships. Is there anything that you would say was more significant than others?

Dr. Ingela Schnittger: I make an effort to personally, really connect with my patient who goes to surgery. They have confidence in me, confidence in the decision to go to surgery. I never tell anybody that they have to have surgery. It's a joint decision. I inform the patient about the risk and the benefit. I informed them about what to expect. We talk about the recovery, the recovery after surgery, the surgical procedure. It takes six weeks to just recover from being a surgical patient, but then you have to build up your stamina. I recommend cardiac rehab. Some people can do it on their own, but some people really like the comfort and the support of a cardiac rehab facility and I tell them, if they have endothelial dysfunction, they're going to have pain, that it will be milder, but I will help you with it. We have medication for it. The myocardial bridge will not grow back. There could be some scar tissue there, but it's not going to push on the vessel. Inform the patient, comfort them, reassure them.

You talk about the recovery, which is at least six weeks from surgery. If it's a sternotomy you won't be sitting as the front seat passenger right away, you'll just lay low for a bit, okay? And then you start cardiac rehab at six or seven weeks and you do that for a month. I would say it takes four or five months to build up your stamina to sort out any kind of chest discomfort and treatment for that. And you stay positive, don't go back to work too early, because some people have sort of a stressful, busy kind of a work and they come back to it and their co-worker says, well, now you're fixed, we can just work you to death. Okay, no, no, no, no, don't go back to work too early, take your time, you'll get sick if you go back too early, okay? Be patient.

I have a pep talk, okay? I think you know, as I said, many of our patients, they come from across the country and I make sure to tell them that I will help them for several months after surgery, with prescriptions, with medications, with reassurance, because their local cardiologists may be hesitant or intimidated or not know what to do when they develop their spasm episodes. I think it's critical they know where they are in their recovery. Eventually, they'll graduate to their local doctors, but I'm very careful to discuss this.

JH: You've done an incredible job of explaining the bridges and the degrees and the understanding in so many ways, much better than I expected. But there's one more thing about you. What do *you* do with all the stress and all the work that you've got? How does Dr. Ingela Schnittger unwind, relax, enjoy? What do you do when you're not working with the healthcare team?

Dr. Ingela Schnittger: I don't know, I guess I have to admit I don't have one single hobby that I engage in. I do work a lot. I mean, I often end up reading or writing from home on the weekends. I like to exercise. I have my own gym. I try to exercise every day, or at least five days a week. I go hiking if I'm out of town. I like to travel. I have family in Europe. As you may have understood, I'm born and raised in Sweden. I still have family there, and family in France, so the pandemic put a dent in that, but I like to spend time with family and visit them. I'm not a gardener, but I guess that's always there if you think that you are going to retire one day. It's like, oh my God, what am I going to do? But I'm not there yet. I love my job. As long as you enjoy what you're doing, you keep doing it right?

JH: If there were one thing you would like to leave the audience with for those of us who are really engaged in taking notes on some of the things that you said, what would it be?

Dr. Ingela Schnittger: On this topic of chest pain, I would say don't give up. If you have chest pain and if you have not gotten an explanation for it and perhaps, some testing to support the doctor's suspicion and then hopefully some treatment. If you have GERD (acid reflux) and you get a PPI (proton pump inhibitor) and you get better, well that's great, right? But if you have chest pain and you don't get better, you don't get a diagnosis with a treatment, then maybe start to think, "Can this be a myocardial bridge?"

Another thing that I always ask my patients is, "Do you have any family history of heart disease?" And then they tell me about valves and fibrillation and this and that. I say "Did anybody have a heart attack?" "Yeah, my father had a heart attack at age 38." I say uh-uh, that's not normal. And I ask for family history, because if a family member has had what I call premature heart attack, then I suggest this may be something that is afflicting you too, because you know that runs in families. I have father, son, mother, daughter as patients. I have clusters of families where the kids end up having the same problem as the parents. We have tried to look at what's the genetic pattern for inheritance and we couldn't nail it down to one gene, but there are really clusters in various families. So, if you have been diagnosed with the bridge and your 13-year-old son comes to his dad and says, "I get chest pain when I run track," don't just pat them on the back and say, "Honey, don't run so fast,"—because he may have the same problem you had.

DR. JEFFREY FOWLER:
Go Ahead, Provoke Me

(A detailed discussion of the provocative test.)

This chapter, we meet interventional cardiologist, Dr. Jeffrey Fowler. I want to be very certain to mention that this is a chapter for patients and doctors as well. Dr. Fowler will be discussing the process and the necessity for the provocative test to help alleviate the uncertainty of whether or not the bridge is causing symptoms. This chapter continues the journey from initial diagnosis to proper testing to surgery. With Dr. Fowler's generous support, we're going to learn the details of the provocative testing we've been hearing so much about.

Dr. Jeffrey Fowler is an interventional cardiologist and is board certified in General Cardiovascular disease and interventional cardiology by the American Board of Internal Medicine. His medical degree is from Lake Erie College of Osteopathic Medicine, and he completed his residency at Cleveland Clinic. He is currently Program Director for the Interventional /Structural Cardiology Fellowship program at University of Pittsburgh Medical Center Heart and Vascular institute and Assistant Professor of Medicine at the University of Pittsburgh. He holds other board certifications, Professional memberships, has been published, speaks professionally and is involved in on-going research projects.

Jeff Holden (Host): The provocative test. We hear about it, we talk about it. A lot of people have explained it as it was for them, but many people just know the words. They don't really know what takes place or how it's done so we're really going to benefit a lot of readers and I suspect a lot of doctors as well, when we finally get to this firsthand understanding of the significance of this testing, this provocative testing. Dr. Fowler, who is it that does this testing?

Dr. Jeffrey Fowler (Guest): There are multiple different subspecialties within cardiology. Most people think you just go to a general cardiologist, but within cardiology we have imaging specialists who focus on particular aspects of the cardiac imaging modalities we use. We have electrical cardiologists that focus on the different rhythm challenges and procedures related to that, and an interventional cardiologist is a cardiologist that has additional training in minimally invasive catheter-based procedures. Most of your audience is probably familiar with a stent that's placed in the coronary artery in the setting of, say, a heart attack or chest pain that somebody may have. That's done by an interventional cardiologist. These minimally invasive procedures are done with catheters placed in either arteries or veins using small wires, small balloons, small stents. We also do diagnostic procedures where we use certain medications and different tools to evaluate the pressure and flow in the coronary arteries, which becomes particularly important in an intramyocardial bridge.

JH: I want to make sure it's clear even though the interventional cardiologist does the stents, it does not mean every patient is getting a stent. If you're working with an interventional cardiologist, it's really all part of the process, done properly, in my opinion. They know that the discovery of the myocardial bridge is best done non-invasively, through a CT angiogram and with contrast of course, since that's the first step. I'm sure you also review the CT to confirm the nature of the bridge before you suggest moving on to the provocative test. Could you tell us what's important to ask when getting that CT angiogram and give us an overview of it when somebody's starting their journey to diagnosis?

Dr. Jeffrey Fowler: Yes. A coronary CTA is an important non-invasive sort of anatomical assessment of the coronary arteries. A lot of these patients may not even know they have a myocardial bridge. They present typically with chest pain, and so part of the evaluation of chest pain includes usually starting with non-invasive testing to assess their chest pain. Those can be either anatomical tests, like a coronary CTA, where we actually look at the blood vessels and we're looking for things like atherosclerotic or cholesterol plaques. We're looking at the origin and course of the coronary artery. We're looking for abnormalities in the coronary artery, like a myocardial bridge. Other patients may get non-invasive testing, like stress tests, which look at functional assessment of the coronary arteries.

If a patient has a myocardial bridge either diagnosed on a catheter originally or there's some concern for it, we order a coronary CTA for that specific reason, we want to make sure that we're fully evaluating that myocardial bridge. A coronary CTA is a special type of CAT scan that does give contrast. It's a gated CT scan, which means that it is timed with the cardiac cycle, coronary arteries fill in diastole or the resting phase of the heart, and we want a high-resolution scan that can split off the systolic phase and the diastolic phase of the heart so we can look at when the coronary arteries fill. The whole cardiac cycle is also helpful on a coronary CTA because the imager can look at that whole cardiac cycle and look at both systole when there's often compression with a myocardial bridge and then diastole and make a comment about the systolic compression that occurs in a coronary CTA. The other aspects of a bridge that we're looking at are the length of the bridge and the depth of muscle that's overlying the artery. There are lot of important aspects of a coronary CTA that can help to identify the bridge and important parts of the bridge.

JH: We know that there could be as many as one in four people with a myocardial bridge. Obviously, 25% of the population is not symptomatic. If somebody presents with chest pain that doesn't seem appropriate for their particular health, lifestyle, et cetera, why would a cardiologist not start with this to rule out a bridge immediately?

Dr. Jeffrey Fowler: Well, as you mentioned, there are a lot of patients who have bridges that are asymptomatic, and when we're evaluating chest pain, a myocardial bridge is not the most common cause of a chest pain syndrome. Most cardiologists are dealing with patients who have some characteristic of their chest pain that is considered classic for blockages, which may be an exertional chest pain. They may have other risk factors for atherosclerosis, like high blood pressure and high cholesterol, and their age plays a role and so the atherosclerotic plaques or blockages are the most common cause of chest pain so most cardiologists do start with either a functional assessment, such as a stress test, to look for the blood flow in the heart arteries as a first step, and then oftentimes, if there's some concern on that, they'll move on to an anatomical assessment with either a coronary CTA or potentially be moving directly to a heart catheterization. So, while a lot of your audience is particularly attuned to a myocardial bridge as one of the causes for chest pain, from my practice that is not the most common cause of chest pain that I see on a day-to-day basis or in most patients.

JH: One thing we see often: Let's say, you go to the hospital where you're presenting with chest pain, you're concerned. Quite often they'll do an angiogram right away, prior to the CT. Why would they do the invasive test first versus the CT first?

Dr. Jeffrey Fowler: It really depends on how the patient presents, what their symptoms are, how convinced you are that there is some abnormality that may need an intervention. If they're having ongoing damage or a heart attack that's going on, moving directly to an invasive study is the appropriate next step. A coronary CTA does have its limitations. We talked about some of the strengths of what it can identify in the bridge, but as cholesterol plaques calcify in the arteries, that calcification sometimes makes it very difficult to know what's on the outside of the vessel versus what's actually encroaching on the lumen and decreasing blood flow to the heart muscle. Some of the calcium just obscures the view of the vessel. There are a lot of reasons why an invasive cath may be the first step for someone. It really depends on their symptoms, their presentation, our concern level, those types of things.

JH: I can appreciate now, then, why you might go to that extreme first. So now the patient is fortunate or unfortunate enough to have been diagnosed. We know they're symptomatic, we know something's going on. You've got your CT. It then progresses to that next step for those hospital systems and cardiologists that are looking to want to understand what's happening a little bit more in detail. So now they're going to say, okay, this provocative test, and I know even in my case and in many situations from people that we speak with that provocative testing is not the first line of thought in many cardiologists' minds simply because their system may not do it or they may not be that familiar with it. We were at wit's end in my situation: the cardiologist, the electrophysiologist, everybody who was working on my case said "We have no idea, we don't know what to do with you." They suggested one more test, because I had severe vasospasms. "You present well, you're clean, there's no clogged arteries, everything looks great. Maybe you just need to get this particular test." I didn't realize only a handful of hospitals in the country did the testing and one was in my backyard. I was fortunate to be able to be referred to Stanford.

How do you prepare the patient for what's going on and what you're going to be able to identify through this provocative test?

Dr. Jeffrey Fowler: In that scenario, it's not uncommon once a myocardial bridge is identified, say on a coronary CTA, and you have some number of symptoms associated with it, to do an empiric trial of medications, and some of that's a risk benefit sort of analysis. When we talk about doing a provocative test, we're talking about moving on to an invasive procedure with manipulation of certain medications to change the dynamics in the heart to make a diagnosis. However, there's some amount of risk with that as well, and so a lot of patients respond very well to an empiric treatment of medications that can help to reduce their symptoms. I think when we're really unsure what's going on and they're either not responding to an empiric treatment of medication or, in the case we're going to talk about a little later today, there are some patients who are very adamantly against taking medications without having an established diagnosis that we move on to an invasive test that can help to establish a diagnosis, and so when that's the case, we move on then to the heart catheterization. And when we do this heart catheterization, most of the times at this point we know that atherosclerosis is not the driving concern here. We've seen on the coronary CTA they have no coronary calcium, there is no atherosclerotic burden, and we're really looking to identify the other causes of chest pain that are often overlooked or sometimes not even assessed for because, as you mentioned, certain systems don't have the ability to do that or maybe even some of the understanding of how to get that accomplished.

When I bring someone in for that type of provocative testing or physiologic testing, I usually prepare them by first describing what's going to happen. I bring them into the cath lab the day of the procedure and we talk about what's going to happen during their heart catheterization. I will enter the artery either in their wrist, the radial artery, their groin, or in the femoral artery. We sterilize and place sterile dressings down on them. I give them some light sedation to help to relieve some pain and anxiety, but they're still going to be for the most part, awake. We want them breathing on their own, we want to be able to talk to them. If we need to, we will provide numbing medication over the site that we're going to be entering and we enter that artery, like I said, either in the wrist or the groin. We then put catheters up into the arteries and we take pictures with contrast dye of the arteries. After we take those initial set of pictures, then we start to work through an algorithm where we assess the different causes of chest pain.

One of those causes you mentioned may be endothelial dysfunction or vasospasm. We will do a full assessment of the microvasculature of the heart and understand if there's any dysfunction there and then if there is a concern for a bridge, we'll go on and do physiologic testing and perhaps even intravascular imaging of the bridge as well.

JH: You mentioned, we're awake, which I recall vividly, and for anybody who's thinking, this is a painful procedure, you really don't feel much. You have us pretty well sedated and comfortable. I will suggest it is a bizarre procedure when we are actually talking to you as you're in our hearts doing things and we recognize things happening. The next part of that is you use a chemical that's, from what I understand, not so easy to get hold of: acetylcholine, but it's a chemical that's found naturally in our system. It controls muscle contraction and by inserting that into the artery itself, how it responds is what dictates the severity of dysfunction. Correct?

Dr. Jeffrey Fowler: Yes, for vasoreactivity or looking for vasospasm in an artery, we'll start with the acetylcholine provocative test. This is specifically looking for endothelial dysfunction and vasospasm. You're right, while this is a naturally occurring substance in the body, getting it in a pharmaceutical form that we can then deliver into the coronary is a little bit challenging. It actually is a formulation derived from eye drops, acetylcholine eye drops, that the pharmacy helps to create a stock solution of that's been diluted down that we can use to inject into the coronary artery. Acetylcholine works on the inner lining or the endothelium of the artery. In a normal endothelium there's a chemical process that occurs when, in response to acetylcholine, it releases nitric oxide which dilates the artery. However, in a dysfunctional artery, we often see we don't have that nitric oxide response. Instead we have a smooth muscle contraction response, which also occurs with acetylcholine, and we get a vasospastic response. If somebody has a normal, intact endothelium with no propensity towards vasospasm, the escalating doses of acetylcholine that I introduced in the coronary artery will cause no change to the caliber of the coronary artery. But if there is either endothelial dysfunction or significant vasospasm with even some of the lower doses of acetylcholine we use, we immediately see that artery clamp down and the blood flow reduced to the heart muscle and often that's associated with symptoms like chest pain. I see EKG changes on the monitor that I'm monitoring with, so it often can be quite dramatic.

JH: I can attest to the drama of that because it got to the point where I was like, that's the symptom and it's really severe and I recognize it right now.

Immediately the antidote was inserted which I'll let you explain as well for somebody who's fearing this testing. If the thing starts to clamp down, what do you do to fix it once you've stuck the stuff in there?

Dr. Jeffrey Fowler: Luckily, we do have the ability to reverse the acetylcholine with nitroglycerin. We then inject a good dose of nitroglycerin into the artery, which will then vasodilate the artery and relieve the symptoms and the changes that we see. While we're doing this, there's very close monitoring of the heart rhythm on the EKG, the chest pain symptoms, the hemodynamics meaning blood pressure, as well as the angiogram that's looking at the response that the artery is having, and we have the ability very quickly reverse any spasm that may be occurring. So once the diagnosis is made, we don't just let the patient sit there with the spasm and the pain. We immediately reverse it, dilate the artery, symptoms resolve and we now have a diagnosis, or at least part of a diagnosis, there.

JH: That's the beauty of being communicative. When you're on the table, it's like, yeah, this is hurting, this is the pain, this is what the sensation is, and you've been able to re-create it and then negate it.

Dr. Jeffrey Fowler: Some of those concerns get addressed ahead of time too. When I do a procedure like this, I try to go step-by-step with the patient before the procedure about what medications they're going to be using, what the responses are that we may anticipate with these medications and how we'll handle those, to try to just relieve some of that anxiety as well that these are controlled settings. We're doing this in a very stepwise fashion. We have the ability to take care of what happens in there.

JH: And to emphasize, the use of the chemical, the proper use of the chemical, the understanding, the skillset on how to relieve the symptom, this is a trained skill. This isn't something somebody's going to come into and start attempting to do on their own in a system that thinks they can do a provocative test. It's quite a sophisticated procedure and in a myocardial bridge situation you may or may not have an endothelial dysfunction. So you may find people whom you do this test on and everything works fine, even though they are having a symptomatic bridge, correct?

Dr. Jeffrey Fowler: Right. Vasospasm and endothelial dysfunction often go hand-in-hand with bridges. We often see them together. But when we are assessing for the physiologic significance of a coronary bridge, what we're really looking to see is how impactful is the systolic compression of that muscle in the artery, especially as you elevate your heart rate into what it would be in an exertion. That's yet another part of the test. We may start with the acetylcholine provocative test to assess the endothelium to see if there's also spasm as part of the problem that's going on. Then, we also will move on in a bridge and do special physiologic testing with yet another medication called dobutamine. Dobutamine is an inotropic medication that works on the beta receptors of the heart to speed up the heart rate and increase the force of contraction, and by giving escalating doses of dobutamine I can drive a patient's heart rate up into a range that they would see when they're, say, exercising. In fact, in order to get a diagnostic test, my goal is to reach 85% of their peak predicted maximal heart rate, and so if I can hit that heart rate goal and they don't have a drop in their blood flow, then that bridge is really not physiologically significant for them. If at any point prior to hitting that 85% goal we see a significant drop in the blood flow from that bridge, then we know that systolic compression, the decrease in the diastolic filling time or the relaxation filling time of the vessel is causing a decrease in blood flow to the heart artery and that's a significant bridge.

JH: I'll share again in that process and the procedure, as the dobutamine is being entered, it's almost as if the interventional cardiologist is speaking to you, as if you are the recipient of a gas pedal and "okay, we're going to accelerate your heart. This is going to feel a little bit awkward." It's one of the most bizarre sensations to be laying still and have your heart racing as if you were running up a hill and just feel the sensation of the movement and upward in terms of the heart rate, to the point where you know it reaches its desired beats per minute, and then you start to back it off again, just as if you were stepping on the brakes. Right, for the people who are listening and about to undergo a provocative test. It's all intentional, it's understood and you're in great hands. It's just going to feel very, very strange as you go through the process.

Dr. Jeffrey Fowler: Yes, it's a bizarre feeling to feel like you're exercising while you're laying flat on your back on the table.

JH: There are some people who would like that and think, hey, can I lose weight while I'm laying here? Can I find a way to do this?

Why do you think there's only a handful of healthcare systems that do this provocative testing? Do you see more and more acceptance of learning and using the testing?

Dr. Jeffrey Fowler: I would say there's definitely more and more acceptance and learning and growth in the field here of assessing for different types of chest pain other than atherosclerotic plaques.

I know your audience is probably familiar with the term ANOCA or angina without obstructive coronary artery disease, and there is definitely growth in this field. However, it is still, for the most part, organized into what I would call centers of excellence. These tests are highly specialized tests. They require some specific equipment and software and pressure wires or flow wires we're using to assess the blood flow in the heart arteries. It also takes time and specialized medications and specialized observation of the patient, ability to reverse what's going on, and so, as you can imagine, you want that expertise to be centralized in areas that do these frequently, that see these patients on a regular basis and are comfortable with these things. So, there is definitely growth in this field and I think that there will continue to be growth in this field and it will become a little bit more ubiquitous. There are still centers of excellence that will likely carry the bulk of the volume and be driving this field.

JH: I also want to applaud you. You mentioned ANOCA. I know during the process of a particular patient's testing, you reached out or had communicated with Dr. Shah, who is doing the Yale study, and has been one of our guests. I think the collaboration and the understanding of trying to get some best practices for these procedures for all of us who have the condition are that we just can't do enough of that and, if I'm not mistaken, you communicated with Dr. Tremmel of Stanford as well, correct?

Dr. Jeffrey Fowler: I haven't actually spoken with her directly, but we have reached out to her and she will be coming to Pittsburgh to UPMC to be giving one of our cardiology grand rounds and I have a dinner meeting with her the night before. I am looking forward to picking her brain even more directly during that meeting. Dr. Shah and I are close and we communicate through phone call and text and he certainly is one of the leaders in this field, along with Dr. Tremmel as well. They have helped to grow the knowledge in this field, both in some of the research they're doing and some of the protocols they're developing. While we are developing our own practice, it's not uncommon for me to reach out to Dr. Shah or Dr. Tremmel or some of the others in this field and say, hey, I got a really interesting case. Here's how I was going to tackle it. How would you tackle it?

In the particular case, which we're going to talk about in a little bit, I was actually going to do some of the bridge testing first and then finish with the provocative testing, Dr. Shah made a comment that he likes to do the acetylcholine provocative testing first before the wire is introduced, because the wire itself can cause some vasoconstriction. I thought that was a wonderful recommendation and so I think, right before we started the procedure, I may have mentioned to the patient that I was going to change the order up a little bit from my discussion with him in the preoperative period. I think he understood the rationale for it as well and trusted us to move forward with it.

JH: I know this patient and he is quite the research-oriented individual with a very strong opinion on how he wants things done. He's certainly one of those characters who would have said "No, I don't want the medication, just skip the medication part. I'm happy, I'm authorizing you to go ahead and do the provocative test on me and let's figure out what's going on." I think that's a good point to discuss the procedure in his case. He's given us the permission to use his report as an example. Would you now walk us through what it looked like going through his provocative testing?

Dr. Jeffrey Fowler: As you mentioned, this patient came to us with a myocardial bridge that was seen on a coronary CTA. At the point that he was referred to us, we were at the stage where we were recommending proceeding forward with an invasive coronary angiogram, the heart catheterization, with all of the provocative and physiologic testing. The catheter that's been inserted into his radial artery, coming down his aorta and cannulating his left main coronary artery, there's contrast dye going into his arteries and lighting up the lumen of his arteries. His arteries are large. There are no blockages inside the arteries. They look normal for the most part, because this is a 3D structure. An x-ray is a 2D modality. We take these pictures in multiple different views, and as you watch the contrast dye go in and you watch the heart beating, you can appreciate maybe the caliber of the artery becomes compressed when the heart actually squeezes and we call that dynamic systolic compression.

With each systole or each squeeze of the heart, the muscle overlying the LAD is squeezing some of the contrast dye and therefore some of the blood out of that artery and compressing that artery. Now, as we discussed, the arteries fill predominantly during diastole or during the relaxation phase, and so oftentimes there's no symptoms at rest because even though there is some amount of compression with each systole or each contraction, because it fills during diastole, the blood flow to the rest of the heart muscle or the myocardium is still preserved at rest. When you exert yourself and you increase your force of contraction in the heart rate and then you decrease the amount of diastole or filling time that the coronary arteries have, we can then see a drop off in the blood flow to the distal vessel and that's what marks a hemodynamically significant myocardial bridge. So, as you mentioned, there are a lot of patients who have bridges that are not hemodynamically significant and are unlikely the cause of their chest pain. But if we can prove that at elevated heart rates and force of contraction this blood flow is decreased to the heart muscle, then that is the most likely cause of their chest pain in a bridge.

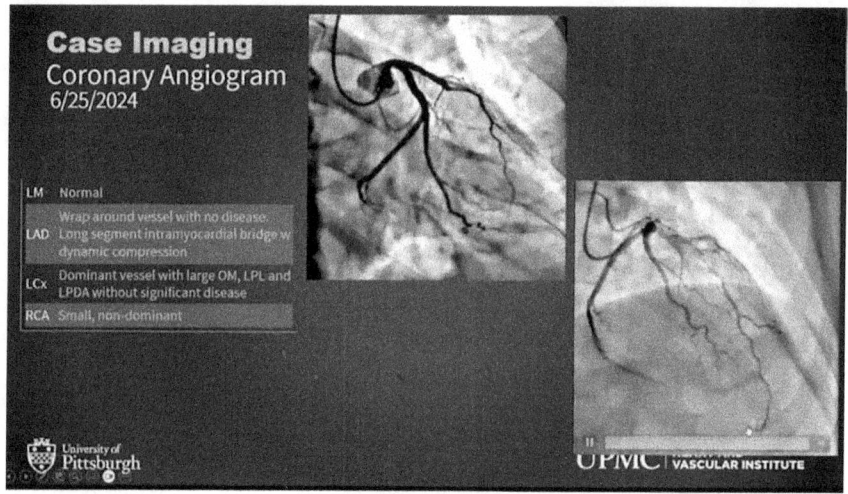

The next phase of the test, as I mentioned, we went to the acetylcholine provocative testing.

The baseline angiogram is for reference and we're going to keep our eye on the LAD vessel. I first gave him a test dose of just 10 micrograms of acetylcholine just to see how he'll tolerate it, and he tolerates it well, without any concerns. Then I go on to the provocative dose, which is 100 micrograms of acetylcholine and you may be able to appreciate there is a slight decrease in the diameter or the caliber of the artery, especially just after the bridge, sort of in the segment by the branch, this diagonal branch, and that does indicate that he does have a little bit of endothelial dysfunction associated with this bridge, but a diagnosis of vasospasm would require that this artery constricted down to less than 90% of what it was in its original caliber.

We have just a little bit of constriction, which is some evidence of some endothelial dysfunction, but not vasospasm.

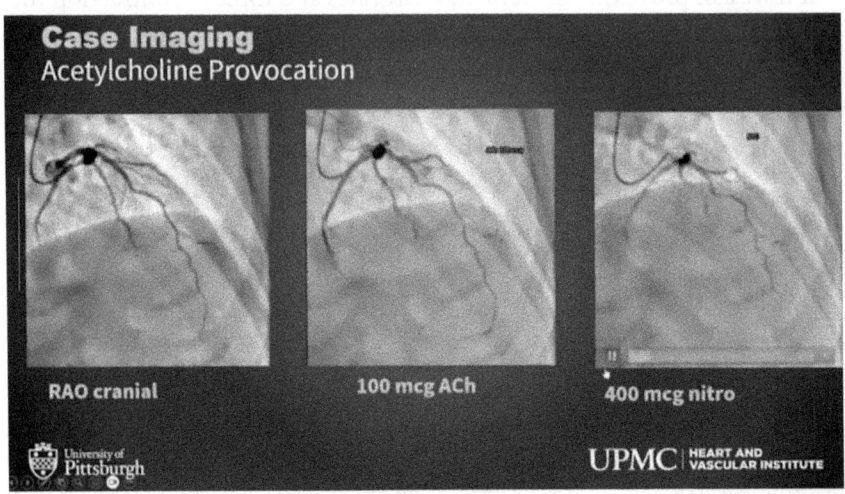

JH: And if I could ask just a quick question there on the endothelial dysfunction, there is some assumption that the compression, the beating that artery takes is sometimes what causes it to dysfunction? It's been getting beat up for so long that it doesn't open up as much as it should, even in the resting phase of the heartbeat, so it doesn't fill as well as it should. And on top of the endothelial dysfunction, with the compression for the vasospasms you have a compounding effect of cascading pain in some cases, or ischemia, correct?

Dr. Jeffrey Fowler: Absolutely, that's absolutely correct and that's why it's important to assess this part of the test as well. You know, with the endothelial dysfunction, the vasospasm, with the bridge, could create a severely endothelial dysfunctional situation.

As we had mentioned earlier, we then reverse the acetylcholine agent and now his arteries are back to the normal caliber they were before the acetylcholine went in. That's an important part of the provocative test. Then we'll move on to the next phase of the test. This is the dobutamine challenge that we talked about. We insert a special pressure wire with a pressure sensor as a surrogate for flow, down the artery and we measure at baseline the flow at the catheter and at the pressure sensor in the middle of the artery, past his myocardial bridge and at baseline, he has normal flow through this myocardial bridge. We then start giving him escalating doses of dobutamine and what we're trying to do is get a decrease in the ratio of blood flow or the pressure ratios from before the bridge and after the bridge less than 0.76. This number shows the decrease in blood flow from before the bridge and after the bridge at escalating doses of dobutamine. And when we hit 130 beats per minute, which is well under his 85% of peak maximal heart rate, his bridge became hemodynamically significant at 0.69. So I didn't need to drive him up to 140, 150 beats per minute, which would be sort of that, that 85% mark. Because even at 130 beats per minute which, as you can imagine, someone as active as he is, he hits that heart rate target probably fairly quickly with his exertion. We can see a drop in the blood flow across that bridge.

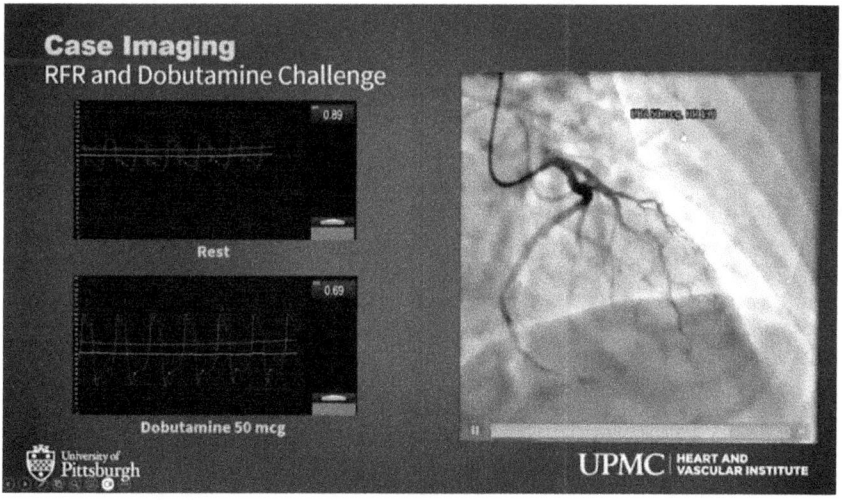

JH: Therefore, you're symptomatic and pain presents itself.

Dr. Jeffrey Fowler: At this point we can say he definitely has a drop in blood flow across that bridge at a heart rate of 130. And so, given his exertional symptoms and the lack of all of the other causes of his chest pain, that this is the cause. Before we say the bridge is the only cause of it, we do go on and we do further testing. We tested his microvasculature as well. So that same pressure wire has a temperature sensor. What we do is we take small aliquots of cold saline, three milliliters of cold saline and I inject the cold saline down the coronary artery and I measure the mean transit time of the cold saline down the artery at rest. And then I give him a vasodilator medication, yet another medication. This one is called adenosine, and adenosine will dilate all of the microvasculature and all of the arteries of the heart so I can then look at the mean transit time of that cold saline when the arteries are fully dilated. That should increase the mean transit time because we're getting increased flow through the arteries, and that difference of the rest flow compared to the fully hyperemic or fully dilated flow is called your coronary flow reserve. It's your ability, your heart's ability, to increase the coronary flow reserve by dilating the arteries in response to an increased need, such as exerting yourself.

There are patients who have coronary microvascular dysfunction, where their microvasculature cannot dilate appropriately in response to a demand like an exertion, and therefore they get chest pain from microvascular dysfunction. The coronary flow reserve should be greater than two, and so that's a flow ratio that increases greater than essentially double of what is at rest. His is robustly normal at 3.2. If his coronary flow reserve were less than two, then on top of his bridge we would also diagnose that he has some dysfunction of his microvasculature and the ability for his microvasculature to appropriately dilate in response to an increased demand and exertion. Because that wire also can assess pressure, looking at the ratio of the flow based on the transit times and the pressure, we can also calculate his resistance in the artery. So this is the IMR, or the index of microvascular resistance. This should be less than 25 in a normal scenario. He has normal coronary flow reserve with normal resistance so this confirms that his microvasculature is normal. He does not have coronary microvascular dysfunction.

Now at the end of his testing, we have really identified very important aspects of his chest pain. Number one, we know he has no atherosclerotic plaques or cholesterol plaques that are causing a decrease in blood flow in the heart artery. We tested with a provocative test in acetylcholine for vasospasm and while he does have some mild endothelial dysfunction associated with his bridge, he does not have vasospasm. The microvasculature is robustly normal in his coronary flow reserve and his microvascular resistance. And with the dobutamine challenge of his bridge we do indeed see a decrease in blood flow at a heart rate of 130 beats per minute. That's consistent with ischemia, or decreased blood flow with the dobutamine across that bridge. These are all confirmatory that he has really no other cause for his chest pain than this positive intramyocardial bridge.

I went one step further and we did intravascular imaging of his myocardial bridge. This is a movie of intravascular ultrasound. This is an ultrasound catheter that's placed inside of the artery over the wire. This is the inside of the artery so you can see the layers of the artery around the wire, around the catheter that the ultrasound is using sound waves to identify. Overlying the artery there is an echo-lucent or black, dark sort of crescent moon shaped structure. That is his muscle band. That's overlying that artery and compressing that artery.

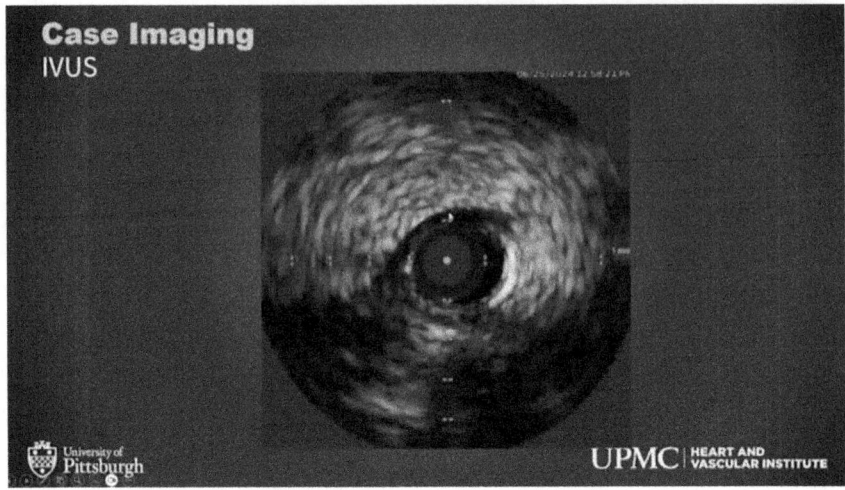

Dr. Jeffrey Fowler: That's really the totality of his testing, where we went from looking at the diagnostic coronary angiogram, doing vasoactive testing with acetylcholine for spasm, we assessed the microvascular, we assessed the physiology of the bridge and the blood flow and even did intravascular imaging of the bridge. With all of that information we can then package that together and send that to his surgeon and we can sit down together and evaluate this testing and talk with the patient about what the next steps for treatment would be for him.

JH: We see IFR (instantaneous wave-free ratio) and FFR (fractional flow reserve) and DFFR (diastolic fractional flow reserve). Is there significance to these or relevance to what you just walked us through?

Dr. Jeffrey Fowler: Those modalities are very similar to what we're doing. When we're assessing an atherosclerotic plaque in, say, the main artery, we use the same type of pressure wires looking at the flow before and after a blockage, similar to how we would in a myocardial bridge. We can use certain hyperemic or vasodilating agents to look at the flow across them as well. We also can look at just the diastolic phase of the cardiac cycle to look at the flow across it, and so that's where we get the different indices that we're looking at. Some are what we call non-hyperemic or without a vasodilating agent, looking at just the diastolic phase. Some are a full hyperemic, meaning a vasodilator agent was given and we're looking at the flow across that blockage. In that sense, it's the same sort of technology.

The difference, then, is we're now using certain medications to manipulate the artery and look for provocative testing with the vasospasm, using the dobutamine to speed up the heart rate and look at what those physiologic flows are at different heart rates or different levels of exertion. Even this intravascular ultrasound that I talked about, the imaging we often will use with this tool when we place the stent, is to assess how our stent has expanded. Is it opposed to the vessel? Is it large enough, what the size of the vessel is, to grow the stent to the appropriate size? And so all of these tools are used in other cases as well, but have specific indications in working up this type of chest pain.

JH: And I think for the novice to be bantering around a lot of those terms is maybe a little over all our heads. We just need to know are we hemodynamically significant in the outcome?

Dr. Jeffrey Fowler: To be honest with you, a lot of the different alphabet soup of IFR, RFR, DFR, are somewhat developed as each company who provides these wires and makes these wires, come up with their own sort of proprietary algorithms and how to assess pressure and flow, identify them with a different terminology. There's proprietary software that helps to determine what the flow is. So that's where a lot of these different terms IFR, DFR, RFR come from. They're really all testing a very similar thing. They're testing the flow from a proximal portion of the artery, either at the guide catheter and then past the blockage at the transducer of the wire and then where they're looking at that flow and whether they're using a hyperemic agent like adenosine or using just a portion of the cardiac cycle with diastole. That's sort of how we get all these different variations on the same theme. We could spend a lot of time going through each one of those and how each company sort of developed their specific pressure wire and what they're looking at, but they're all testing a very similar concept.

JH: My head already hurts from the explanation.

You live and work in an extremely stressful environment. I know as patients, we like to interview and speak with the people who are going to be working on our bodies and we wonder what do you do for fun? How do you relax? What's a little bit of the personal side of Dr. Fowler look like?

Dr. Jeffrey Fowler: Yeah, of course. The job can be stressful whenever you're dealing with patient's health and doing these procedures. I like to relax with my family. I'm married and have three kids, 16, 14, and 12. They're very active in different sporting events specifically, and so I spend a lot of time at baseball fields and softball fields and hockey rinks and doing fun things with them. I also like to exercise. I'm a big runner and do some biking as well and some resistance training. Those are the best ways for me to unwind. Being active, being with family, friends, loved ones, trying to keep perspective on what's going on and try to untangle some of the stress sometimes.

JH: Having three, almost, teenagers I can understand you'll have your hands full for a period of time.

How about any final words to leave with our readers? I know your procedures now in the hospital at UPMC are changing to where you're taking on different cases. You're looking at things a little bit differently. We're trying to establish somebody in every state where we can say here's a quality institution so please tell us what's happening there in Pennsylvania.

Dr. Jeffrey Fowler: As I mentioned, the most common cause of chest pain is still atherosclerosis, and so oftentimes patients get to cardiologists and get testing, even invasive testing, looking specifically for atherosclerosis, and that often is the cause of their chest pain. But there is another whole group of patients who do not have any atherosclerosis but still have very real cardiac chest pain, and a lot of these patients, after they go through a cath that shows no blockages, are told oh, your chest pain is non-cardiac, it's not associated with your heart. And that may not necessarily be true. So what we're developing here has been developed at many other large institutions as well. We're looking at chest pain syndromes that occur for reasons other than atherosclerotic plaques, and we've talked about those today. That could include vasospasm or microvascular dysfunction or intramyocardial bridges, so we have developed a whole team that includes not only some of our non-invasive cardiologists that see the patients, oftentimes initially in the office, or our cardiac imagers, who specialize in reading these coronary CTAs, or interventionalists like myself who can do advanced testing in the cath lab, to even our cardiac surgeons, who can offer unique treatment modalities for these patients.

I think it's really important for a patient who's struggling with chest pain and may be told you don't have blockages so your chest pain is likely not your heart, that maybe that isn't sufficient enough and that until they interact with a center of excellence that has some specialty in evaluating for other causes of this chest pain, you don't know for sure that it's not cardiac. There's a lot of patients who would benefit from this testing and some treatment to try to help relieve this chest pain and improve their outcomes as well so that's what we're doing at UPMC. We're not the only ones and certainly we weren't the first ones. Like I'd mentioned, we talk a lot with a lot of the other institutions that are part of this group. There's a network called the Microvascular Network that you can look up online, where you can look at other institutions that are doing a lot of these sort of protocols or algorithms and testing for other cardiac chest pain that's not from atherosclerosis.

To see the complete video imaging and descriptions in this chapter, visit the YouTube Channel, "Imperfect Heart", episode 44.

DR. MARK FRANCIS BERRY: Permission to Enter

(An explanation of the process of a sternotomy.)

When the prospect of open-heart surgery looms, the heart races with more than anticipation—it's a journey of resilience and precision. Dr. Mark Francis Berry, a Stanford Thoracic Surgeon, walks us through the mysteries of the sternotomy, a procedure that has saved countless lives but is feared, many times, more than the actual heart surgery being performed that precipitated the need for the sternotomy.

From the meticulous dance of the surgical team to the crucial role of post-operative care, this operation is as much about skilled choreography as it is about medical necessity. With more than 500,000 sternotomies performed annually in the United States, it is far from uncommon. It's the ability to humanize the experience, discuss the fears of the patient and the importance of support during recovery, that give this discussion a much more realistic look at the most frequently used procedure to allow complete access to our hearts.

Jeff Holden (Host): Dr. Berry, welcome to Imperfect Heart.

Dr. Mark Berry (Guest): I appreciate being here. Thank you so much for the opportunity to participate.

JH: Let's talk a little bit about some of the observations I've picked up from what listeners to the podcast are telling me. There are over 500,000 sternotomies performed annually and that's, I think, unfortunate. What is it, do you think, that's caused this surgery to become so prolific?

Dr. Mark Berry: I think the reason for those kinds of numbers are two-fold; some good, some bad. One reason is a testament to the fact that the cardiac surgery profession and the surgical and medical profession in general can do very, very complex things very successfully. They can do things for people that in many cases would be leaving people with a deadly condition if it wasn't addressed. It can be done with low morbidity and low chance of dying and with a great chance of returning to your normal quality of life. I think one reason is that there are so many sternotomies done is because it *can* be done. It can be done successfully and there are people who have conditions and who need them. Then the flip side I guess, the not-so-good side, is the fact that so many people need heart surgery or so many people need sternotomy, and sometimes you do a sternotomy because someone has cancer. Along with the sternotomy then, there are some lifestyle things, such as quitting smoking, that you can do that might lower your risk of death from cancer. But there are many things you can't do. You may get it for just bad luck in terms of heart surgery.

There are a lot of lifestyle habits or medical conditions that increase your risk of needing heart surgery, and some are things like smoking or having diabetes, or poorly controlled blood pressure, hypertension. Some things have gotten a lot better in this country, like a lot fewer people smoke, so a lot of cardiovascular disease may be decreasing because there's not as much smoking. On the flip side, there's a bit of a health crisis in our country, in the sense that many people are obese, much more than what you would expect, and that predisposes you to conditions such as hypertension and diabetes, which then predisposes you to things like heart disease, and then that sets you up for potentially needing heart surgery. Going back to the question, why are we doing so many? One is we can do them, and we can do them successfully, which is great. But two, a lot of people need them, which is not so great.

JH: I'm going to make the assumption, since heart disease is the number one killer in the country, that the majority of the sternotomies are heart related.

Dr. Mark Berry: Yes, yes, the overwhelming majority of sternotomies are for some kind of heart surgery procedure.

JH: The second question is, and you can probably answer this better than most, is the sternotomy itself seems to create more fear, anxiety, angst amongst the people who are candidates for heart surgery. In our case the unroofing procedure, and I think part of that's because the understanding of what the sternotomy really is can be misunderstood. People don't know all the details and the ease of access and everything else that it provides the surgeon. Could you walk us through, literally, a step-by-step process once a patient's been prepped? What happens during a sternotomy?

Dr. Mark Berry: Sure. That's a very interesting insight that you have. I actually was thinking about that a little bit when you prepped me for what we would talk about. Before I talk about the steps of the sternotomy, I think the reason why people probably fear that more than actual heart surgery is because it's easier to picture trauma to your body where you break a bone, and it's easy to visualize the scar. It's also easy in your head to think about your chest being opened in this room full of strangers, which can certainly be terrifying, whereas the fact that someone's actually touching your heart and doing something to your heart, that's a little more abstract. Most people have never seen that, so it's harder to say that's terrifying, because it's not something they probably ever thought about before. I think that's probably what it is. That it's easy to picture trauma and the scar and things like that. It's funny because I've seen so many that I don't even think about it, and if someone tells me that they need heart surgery, I don't even think about the approach, whether it's a sternotomy or a minimally invasive surgery or a catheter-based procedure. My thought immediately is to the heart. That's an important organ, maybe the most important. I certainly can understand why people worry about that.

Basically, the steps of a sternotomy are that you obviously bring in a patient to the operating room, the anesthesiology team will safely and very peacefully get those patients to sleep in a very comfortable way, and then there is a whole flurry of activity done to safely do what we call prep, then drape the patient. You set the patient so they're perfectly positioned for anything that might need to be done during the surgery. That includes unexpected developments where, if there are any problems with the heart or bleeding or anything like that, that you're ready to take care of that patient with a really minimal chance that something bad would happen or there'd be a really bad outcome. If you can picture a person needing a sternotomy, they have to be lying back and their head needs to be extended, meaning their chin needs to be up, because you want the sternum to be maximally exposed. What that means for the patient is that they're lying on the operating room table, which is padded, then there's usually what we call a little soft bump under their shoulders so that brings their head back, their chin is as far back as it can go. And we're very careful- actually, and that's one of the more careful things at the beginning of the case, to have the neck extended in a very comfortable way, not overextended, so that they don't wake up with a very stiff neck. You position the patient that way and then you very, very carefully prep the patient in a sterile fashion and then you drape the patient, which is where you expose the part of the chest that needs to be exposed. Then everything else is covered by sterile drapes, so the chance of contamination that could lead to an infection is as minimal as can be.

One of the things that now occurs before any surgery in almost every operating room probably in the world is what they call surgical timeout. That's where everybody in the room is just focused on discussing what the plan is, what all the critical things that need to be done are so everybody's on the same page. A lot of times people think, oh, that's just to make sure you don't do the wrong site surgery or the wrong surgery on the wrong patient, and that's part of it, of course, but the other part is just to get a team of about 10 people focused. We're here for this patient to take care of this. We need all these things, and we need to make sure that they're all available. We need everybody to be ready to do everything that they do. That's a lot of time. So if you're a loved one of a patient, and nowadays you can usually sit in the waiting room and watch an electronic screen that shows what's happening with a patient, for somebody undergoing heart surgery it can be an hour and a half or longer between the time the patient actually goes into the operating room until there's a sign that the surgical team has started the surgery, the actual surgery.

Now, for a sternotomy, you make what we call a midline incision. You make an incision over the top of their sternum, down to the bottom of their sternum, depending on the surgery and depending on what you need access to. That can be way up to the top of your breastbone, your sternum, that you can feel it. Sometimes it can be a little lower so you can kind of hide the scar for some situations. Basically, you cut the skin.

We use what's called a cautery device to go through the soft tissue of the chest, so the subcutaneous fatty tissue, the fascia, which is the leather lining of muscle that holds things together. There's not much muscle actually weighed over your sternum because your pectoralis muscles end just before they reach in the middle, then you get down to the bone itself. There are a lot of important things below the sternum, above the sternum, behind the sternum, and you need to make sure that when you're getting ready to divide the sternum that you protect all those things. You need to make sure that none of the blood vessels above the sternum in your neck or below the sternum near your heart are at risk of being injured when you're dividing the sternum or the breastbone. We use a sternal saw and I think the thing that I often get from patients that they fear the most for any chest injury is this concept of "cracking" the chest.

That just sounds terrible, it sounds painful, but really when the sternum is divided for heart surgery it's a super routine thing. An experienced heart surgeon can probably do it in about three seconds, but it is incredibly precise. The world's possibly most expensive saw is used. It just divides the breastbone. It's a very elegant procedure in the sense where it is a time in the operating room where everybody's taking care of the patient needs to be on the same page, because the anesthesiologists need to stop ventilating the patient, meaning they need to stop filling their lungs up with air so the lungs collapse a little bit, so there's less chance that something could be injured.

When you're dividing the breastbone, the surgeon obviously needs to be laser-focused on what they're doing. Their assistants need to be focused on providing them the exposure, and then the nursing staff needs to be not only giving them the saw but also giving them what they need right afterwards. The sternotomy is probably the quickest part of the surgery, even though it's probably the thing that people fear the most. It's a matter of sawing through the bone and then that's it. There's only slight oozing of blood from the edges of the bone. That's the first step that the surgeons will do. They'll stop that bleeding with cautery and other matters and then they'll put in a sternal retractor.

That again, I think, is something that patients fear the concept of where you're spreading the chest, and that's what the retractor does. But that's what you need. The sternotomy is to give you access to the heart. The retractor holds the bone apart so you can do what you need to do and that's it. That's the sternotomy. And, again, like I mentioned, I think a lot of people fear that, but after that, that's when the real important stuff starts. That's the reason you're there. The problem is with the heart. That's about to be addressed in some way and that's where, really, the expertise of the team and the surgeon come into play.

JH: That's a wonderful description and very well laid out for us to visualize. I have a question for you. As the sternum is being held open with the retractor, where are the arms? Where are our shoulders?

Dr. Mark Berry: In most cases the patients are lying on the bed and they have their arms tucked next to them, so they're just lying by their side.

They're usually wrapped in foam or other comfortable types of material, but their arms are tucked to their side and their shoulders are kind of pulled in close to their chest.

JH: OK, and then what closes it back up once the surgery is complete? How does that process take place?

Dr. Mark Berry: That process involves going through whatever is involved in the primary surgery making sure that everything is okay, making sure everything is functioning appropriately and then it's a matter of bringing the two cut edges of the sternum together. The overwhelming majority of patients who have a sternotomy will have the sternum brought together by putting in stainless steel wires that will bring the two cut edges of the sternum back together. Most patients will probably have eight wires that will be put in the chest. Sometimes, depending on the size of a patient, it may only be seven that are needed on the top part of the sternum. That's the part of the sternum that's called the manubrium. It's just the very top part. If you feel your chest, there's usually a little bit of a slope to that. If you're coming down from your neck down to your lower body, for most people their fingers will come away from their body until it reaches a flat point and then goes flatter.

When we use the sternal wires to close the sternum, we put the wires through the bone in that manubrium, the top part of the sternum, and that's because that's actually a thicker part of bone and you can put the wires through there and they'll hold very, very well. Then lower down in the body of the sternum, oftentimes you'll just put the wires around the edge of the sternum and that's partly because the sternum is more narrow down lower and there is a little bit of a risk that if you put the wires through the sternum it can actually pull through the recovery. For most patients, by putting it around the outside of the bone it will hold it more snug together. So the process is a nicely choreographed team of assistants and surgeon and the scrub tech at the OR table and then the circulating nurse getting all the materials. It's basically putting in all the wires, seven or eight wires through the sternum and then one of the most critical parts of the closure is then pulling everything snug.

You bring the sternal edges back together. The reason that's important is because that essentially closes the chest. When you bring the chest back together that can increase the intrathoracic pressure and if there's anything inside the heart that can get distorted and maybe not function the way it's supposed to, that can display itself in terms of blood pressure or heart rate or other vital signs. Most people have a good habit when they're closing the chest, they tell the anesthesiologist and they tell the room. If something starts to go a little haywire, they know we need to release that pressure and figure out what we need to make sure we didn't change something.

Once you bring the two edges of the sternum together, it's a simple process of just twisting the wires or the edges of the wires around themselves and then clipping the wires. Once you have the edges of the bone nicely snugged together, for most people, we'll push those wires into the edge of the bone. You then close all of the soft tissue above the bone and that's in multiple layers of what we call absorbable suture, the suture that will eventually just go away on its own and for a lot of people it's very skinny. People can often feel the wire, but many people don't even know it's there or ever feel it, and that's the end of it.

JH: I know I was quite disappointed when I went through the airport. I got nothing special. I have these wires in here and nothing. It doesn't set anything off. You want some acknowledgement for what you're carrying in your system and unfortunately you guys do such a good job now with the gauge of the wire that it doesn't set anything off.

The other part that a lot of people are concerned about, obviously, is pain. I think you addressed why the scars are minimal, at this point I barely even notice mine most of the time, and certainly from a distance people wouldn't even pick it up. But pain is the inevitable part of surgery under any circumstance and you have to be prepared and understand that there's going to be some challenges with pain. A lot of the technology has changed today to where the ability to minimize the pain, as the procedure is being taken care of as well as post-surgery, are really significant. Can you walk us through a little bit on some of those techniques now that are capable of minimizing the pain?

Dr. Mark Berry: Yes, that's a super important part of surgery. Good pain control after surgery is important for many reasons. For one, you don't want people to be in pain as they recover because you don't want them to be in pain. But two, it's super important that people are comfortable through their recovery, because that's how you make sure that they recover well with the least chance of complications. If you do a big surgery on somebody and they're in a lot of pain and they're having a hard time getting out of bed or taking deep breaths or coughing, that's a setup for infection such as pneumonia or bedsores or deconditioning, which then sets you up for a longer recovery or more complications. So pain control is super important. For sternotomies, we probably have not made as much progress as maybe many people would hope for this type of thing that's so common. Part of that is because, fortunately, a sternotomy does not hurt as much as other traumatic surgeries, even with all the trauma that I just described with the surgery.

Part of that is that when you close the sternum, you end up with a very stable bone. So, even though it was surgically fractured, when you put the wires in and you bring it together, if it heals well, it's not going to move. What hurts with a broken bone is when the edges of the fracture rub against each other. That's what will cause incredible discomfort and anybody that's broken any bone will know that terrible feeling. When you have a broken bone and you can feel it move, that is, I think, something that people feel a sense of doom because that's not what your body is supposed to be doing. Fortunately for the sternum, once you wire it together, if it's healing well, it doesn't move. It doesn't really hurt as much as other bones and because it's stable, even when people take a deep breath, it doesn't hurt as much. Even a small chest tube incision, which many people have experience with, can be a very tiny incision but can hurt like crazy, even though it's 10 times smaller than the bigger incision. That's because there's muscle there that gets irritated every time you take a deep breath or you cough or you, God forbid, sneeze. That's one of the most violent things you can do and it can really be painful. So fortunately, the sternotomies are not as painful as a lot of other surgeries.

One advance that we have is that people are much more focused on using non-narcotic pain medication to allow them to recover. It used to be we would put them on a strong narcotic pain medicine like oxycodone or Percocet or things that people hear about. But now we'll do what we call multimodality. Most people will need a narcotic pain reliever for a short period of time. Then non-steroidal anti-inflammatories like ibuprofen or Tylenol can be very, very effective for people and with a lot less of the downsides that can come with narcotic pain medicine.

Then there are also what we call nerve medications, like gabapentin or Lyrica (Pregabalin), as a well-known one, or Cymbalta (Duloxetine). Those address pain in a different fashion and they can be much more effective with less downside of the narcotic pain medicines. There have been a lot of different techniques that have been tried. People have tried freezing nerves to try to get them to go numb for a couple months. Occasionally people will put an epidural block in a patient's back to try to numb the nerves at the root to try to keep them from feeling it as they're recovering. There are other pain catheters that can be put in the vicinity of nerves to try to gently infuse pain medicine continuously, just to keep the area numb, and those have had mixed results. Some people, they work great, other people it's hard to tell if they do much more than our standard pain regimen.

JH: I was just saying I had that epidural on both sides, left and right, and, having only experienced it once I don't know if it was better or worse because I don't have anything to compare it to, but I would say that the pain that I had through my procedure was certainly manageable by two days out.

I was able to survive on just the extra strength Tylenol, for all the reasons you mentioned regarding some of the narcotics. Not that it was easy, it wasn't as comfortable as a narcotic might have made it, but it was the preferred choice for me. And once you get through that third, fourth, fifth day, everything gets better for the most part and, to be sure, not linearly better. There are days that are better and days that are not as good as you'd like them to be, but the trend line is all positive. Fear, just fear of all the uncertainty of the procedure is something that everybody deals with in some way, shape or form. As you're going in for a surgery like this, have you seen anything that's worked well to help patients minimize the fear, or things that maybe you've heard from stories that patients have said oh, I just did this and it really helped me accept what was going on.

Dr. Mark Berry: I think there are a couple of things that can be very helpful to people. One thing is being able to give them a very good understanding of, first off, why they need whatever they need, give them a clear but somewhat concise picture of what is going to happen and then what to expect, both in the immediate period after surgery but then in the next month or two as they continue to recover. And I think by just taking away a lot of the unknown, that can often make people feel much, much more comfortable that in their mind, thinking about what it could be or what's involved with it, when they actually have a good, nice, clear explanation, that can, in my experience, make people just a million times more comfortable. And I've seen many patients who come in for an appointment to talk about surgery and you can tell they're just a basket of nerves, that they just haven't slept well, they're super worried. Then to hear about it, it is very sobering. In some cases, you're, well, we're going to stop your heart for a couple hours or for a couple minutes or something, and that's certainly terrifying. But when they hear about the process and the whole thing sounds kind of matter of fact, I think that can put people at ease.

Another thing that's helpful and that I'm very grateful that I have, is having a very good team of people that work with me. That can also provide support to patients, because a lot of times you'll talk to a surgeon for a period of time and you'll talk about a lot and most people will not grasp it all. Fortunately, a lot of people will have their family or their loved ones with them and they're their second set of ears so they can compare notes at the end. It's also very nice that if a patient thinks about something and it wasn't clear to them that they can reach out to the surgeon's team and then have the team members be able to answer their questions in a very reassuring way, and that can also put people at ease. That's important for two reasons; one, it lets them get their questions answered, and it gives them the faith that I'm going to be able to talk to somebody afterwards. They're not just going to cut me loose. I have this whole team of people that are going to help take care of me through the start, through the finish, and that that can be very reassuring for people. Then, things like your podcasts or support groups are oftentimes incredibly helpful to people as well. Sometimes just talking to someone for a couple minutes can really put them at ease and get it from the patient's perspective. A patient may say you know what? It was pretty miserable for the first couple of days, but hey, I'm good now. I got through it and they helped take care of me and it wasn't as bad as I feared, or maybe it was as bad as I feared, but I'm on the other side of it and I would do it again. Those things can be very, very, very helpful for people to just to hear someone say I've been through it. I'm on the other side of what you went through. I had the same fears that you had, and this is what my experience was.

JH: That's a great explanation because it's certainly the fear of the unknown that people are always challenged with and as they get educated and they understand a little bit more, I know for some who are reading, they don't want to know, they don't want to ask that question. I can't stress enough the necessity to advocate for yourself, because you're going to benefit from that, whether it be emotionally or even in the physical healing, to know that no, this is normal, we talked about this, this is okay as you go through it. Obviously, it's the first time for most of us. Did I do something wrong? Did I pop a wire? Should I not have moved out of my zone, so to speak? And I think that leads us into the next part of that, the post-surgical procedure that you as the patient, should really watch. What are some of the things that we have to be careful of once the procedure has been done and now we're working on healing?

Dr. Mark Berry: One is you need to advocate for yourself to make sure you're getting good pain control. And again, going back to the fact that there's no reason to be in pain, we have buckets and buckets and buckets of pain medication in the hospital and in the world and we have many, many different things to do for people. Being comfortable is an incredibly important part of your recovery, because not only for the psychology of being in pain or the fear of having pain, or the fear that if you move you're going to be in pain, but you as the patient are going to recover so much better if you can get out of bed, if you can take deep breaths, if you can cough, if you can sit up in a chair, if you're not just lying in bed and trying not to move, you're going to be back to your normal self a lot faster and you're going to feel better. Being active or being a strong advocate for yourself to make sure that your pain is well controlled, and that can include saying, I don't want to take narcotic pain medicine. I've had a bad reaction to it, or I've had a fear of it, or I know people that have gotten addictions which were credibly disruptive to their life. Those are important too, because you can take those things into account and you can adjust the way you take care of people, because it's not an all, a one or a zero.

It's not like take this pain medicine or you can be in excruciating pain. We can avoid this pain medicine that you fear. May not be perfect, but it'll still good enough that you'll have a good recovery. That's very, very important. Then, when you get discharged from the hospital, I always tell my patients I want you to be as active as possible. Take as many walks as you want. You shouldn't do anything too strenuous until all the bones are healed, because we don't want there to be any healing issues. But the more you do, usually the better you feel and the faster you're back to yourself.

JH: Depression is a part of the healing process, I've learned. Can you speak to that at all? Is there anything familiar to anyone pushing it a little bit more on the mental health side of things? I'm sure patients come to you as well and say, doc, I'm just, I'm miserable, I feel terrible, I don't want to get out of bed. Is there anything you can address to the point of depression?

Dr. Mark Berry: It's an incredibly important topic. I would say that in general, the medical community doesn't do a great job with it. I think the most recognized syndrome that we have is postpartum depression. That took a long time to recognize how important it is and how common it is and how poorly treated it can be. I think there are a lot of reasons for the depression that people can have. One is that you're in the hospital. It's like you're in a fishbowl where you're being watched by so many people and people are coming in all the time. In some ways that can be disturbing to people, especially if you're a private person or you want some quiet. But at the same time, I think it's very reassuring that you can think three days ago my heart was being operated on and I'm connected to all these monitors and people are coming in. If something happens, they're going to find it. Then people go home and they're by themselves and they almost always will have family or a loved one or friends that will be, at the very least, checking in on them. It's a lot quieter and a lot more disturbing. I'm not being watched. What if something is going on? They had me on this monitor for five days. Why did I need it for five days and now I don't need it now? Is there something going on? As you're in your recovery and you're not allowed to do too much, even if we want you to do a lot, we don't want you to be normal in terms of your normal activity. You're not ready for work, your concentration is not going to be back where it needs to be. For a little while, you're alone and maybe people think a little bit about their mortality. Oh my God, I just went through this. What's going to happen to me in the future? Maybe their minds go to what if I'm going to have a complication? Maybe I'm having a complication. Maybe, as you said, maybe I did something and now I broke a wire and now I'm not going to recover as well as I should have, and it's all my fault.

I think that those things all can step to putting people into mental-health issues such as depression or just anxiety, and maybe I simplify it way too much. My treatment is let's get them better, let's tell them they're doing well. If they call us with a problem, don't blow it off, have somebody talk to them, find out what symptoms they're having. Even if it sounds like what this is, is totally normal and I'm going to reassure you that that's normal pain, that having a cough like that is normal. Show the patient that you're taking it seriously enough that you'll look into it. You'll say, well, sounds normal, but let's just get a chest x-ray. Why don't you just go someplace close to home, get the x-ray. We'll get the pictures, we'll take a look, we'll make sure that it's all the way it should be. Or why don't we have a visiting nurse come out and get some blood? Or why don't you just go to the local lab and get some blood work? Let's just check, make sure everything is still on par for recovery. Or, why don't you come in and see our team? The surgeon might be in the operating room, but our nurse practitioner or our physician assistant or somebody else on the team can take a look at things and just make sure that it all looks okay. For me, that's what I usually focus on with people through their recovery is, if they are contacting us with issues, we take it seriously and we try not to just reassure them but also say well, we're going to investigate it and try to reassure you that it really is okay, and if it's not, we'll figure it out and we'll take care of it.

JH: That was a great explanation and to your point, all this activity is going on when you're in the hospital, everything 24-7, and you're checked on, you're wired, you're, everything hooked up, no concerns, because if anything happens, somebody's there to take care of it and all of a sudden you go to the peace and quiet of your home, like instantly, whatever that drive is from point A to point B, and all of a sudden it's quiet. And now you do have that opportunity to think and process what just happened, especially if it wasn't a prepared surgery and it was a sudden heart attack or something that caused you to be opened up for surgery.

That was helpful. I've had four women on the program over the course of this first year. Three of the four have had some sort of issue with their sternal wires having to be removed because they were painful, they could feel them, and two of the four had a sternum non-union. All of it seems fairly easily remedied, although if you're experiencing it you don't know what it is because you only get to do this once in most cases. Can you explain what that is, just for those who maybe experience something like that. Knowing what that is, here's what we do, and it's a very simple process, because all of the three women have all had their wires removed, everything's fine, and two of them had some sort of a plate put on at the top of the sternum and everything's fine. So maybe walk us through what that is that causes it. And they're all small women, they're all fairly petite ladies.

Dr. Mark Berry: So first, just to address the topic of the wires and whether they will ever need to be removed, I would say the overwhelming majority of people don't have any sensation of the wire there, or they don't have an uncomfortable sensation of the wire being present and it doesn't bother them. And the thought of a foreign body in them forever doesn't bother them. But for some people, if they're really skinny, they can feel it and for some people the wire may feel bulkier. It may be a reminder to them of a traumatic experience and that, you know, the scar maybe doesn't bother them because that will oftentimes heal in a much better way than what they fear. But they can still feel this foreign body and I think psychologically sometimes that can be very disturbing for people and sometimes it can hurt. It's sitting there near the edge of your pectoralis muscle and it might irritate it when you're doing things. When they need to be removed, it's not too big of a deal. It requires anesthesia so people are comfortable, but usually just a small incision over the wire and once the bone is healed you don't need the wire anymore. It doesn't have to stay in forever. It's just that it's usually not worth it to take them out for people. We just go in and cut the wire and pull it out. There's, luckily, in my experience, a theoretical risk that something could be injured when you take out the wire and maybe cause some bleeding and then suddenly it's a much bigger deal than anticipated. But for most patients it's just an outpatient procedure and for most of the people that I've had who've had uncomfortable wires, it's usually not all of them, it may just be the ones on the upper part of the chest or some other location that bothers them. I've had a few patients that have had chest surgery and then years later get a condition where they lose a ton of weight and suddenly the wire, which is never an issue for a long time, is suddenly a problem and we'll take them out in those situations as well.

That's the topic of removing wire. Not too big of a deal and if they really bother people they can come out and not too big of a deal to remove them if that's necessary. The sternum and non-union can be a bigger issue. The goal of bringing the sternum together is so the edges of the bone are right up against each other. Hopefully within four to six weeks they've reattached the way any broken bone will, and then, once that happens and it's healed, it's not as strong as what it was before the surgical fracture but it's good enough for anything for almost everybody. And really the key is between the way that you close the breast bone and then the instructions you give patients. You want that bone to heal perfectly the first time. It's one of those get it right the first time types of things. Whereas, if the bone can heal up okay for most people that they're as good as new. For all intents and purposes, what can happen in some people, it can be because maybe they're predisposed to not healing as well if they have things like diabetes or they have other conditions that predispose the poor wound healing.

If the bone doesn't stay together and heal up right away, then you can have a little bit of a gap between the two edges of the sternum. That's what a sternum non-union is. Sometimes that can be because with a little bit of time the wires actually pulled through the bone before the bones actually fused together. That's where the strict sternal precautions that we give people that I'm sure you were lectured on several times, where no push-up type moves, let it be. We don't want to put stress on the bone, we want it just to heal, perfectly the first time.

That's not to say that if someone has a sternal non-union it's because they didn't listen to the sternal precautions. There are all sorts of things that can come into play when that happens and most of them probably have nothing to do with the patient. There's not as much bone to wrap the wires around, so there's a little bit higher chance that the bone, the wire could pull through the bone. That's not the patient's fault, that's not because they didn't follow instructions, it can just be the physics of their body.

The worst kind of consequence of a sternal non-union is that if it gets infected because it didn't heal together, then that's a bit of a mess because that's going to require a little bit more advanced reconstruction procedure, nowhere near the seriousness of heart surgery, but a big deal for sure. The next step is let's hope it doesn't get infected. If it doesn't feel stable to people, they feel a little click when they do things or when they're active, it's uncomfortable and they're not doing what they want to do or they're afraid they're going to hurt it more, that's a big deal too.

That's a case where you know you might need to go back in and close it again. Clean up whatever didn't heal perfectly and then close it again. We try to avoid that because if it didn't heal perfectly the first time, oftentimes the same risk factor for not healing might be the second time. And now you're dealing with something with some scar tissue which is not as healthy as what your original bone was and you may run the risk of it not healing the second time around.

There are things you can do differently. As you mentioned, sometimes you can put a plate on the sternum instead of a wire. There are other types of things that can be used to try to bring the sternum together that are different than wires. That can be different than what was done the first time around, and for most people if something like that happens, it can be fixed in a way that ends up with a good result. Again, you'd like to get it right the first time. You don't want people to have to have this major traumatic event, that it's just a month to three or four months and then they're back to their lifestyle and they're not having to address something else down the line.

JH: The two ladies that had theirs repaired with a plate say they're fine. They said back to normal; they're doing everything they used to do and that was the issue and everything's good.

I want to ask you a question because I think we all get this fear post-surgery. I got COVID two weeks later and it was upper respiratory and I coughed and coughed and coughed and I thought I am absolutely going to destroy everything you put together in there. Can you give us a little bit of assurance that you're not going to cough your wires apart?

Dr. Mark Berry: Even with all the precautions that we give people and we really read them the riot act of not doing anything too strenuous with their sternum, at the same time I'm telling everybody I want you walking an hour a day. I don't want you lying down unless you're actually taking a nap or you're going to sleep for the night. I want you coughing, if there's mucus in your windpipe or in your lung, I want it out because I don't want it to turn into pneumonia. So coughing is okay. It is some cruel twist of fate to give somebody COVID after heart surgery. That's not fair. But your body is going to be able to withstand coughing. We want you to cough. You know we don't want you to be sick with COVID and we don't want you to be coughing violently because of all these things going on. But your sternal closure can tolerate those kinds of things. We want to avoid unnecessary stress. Again, if someone looks like they're trying not to cough, I'm admonishing them, that they're setting themselves up for some trouble. So if you get a cold, you get COVID, you're coughing after heart surgery, it's not going to be the end of the world in almost every case. It's important for people to make sure they stay up with their surgeon and their team of people taking care of them and just make sure everything's okay. For the most part, when you get discharged from the hospital unless there's something really extraordinarily wrong going on you're going to heal well.

JH: I wanted to ask when we were talking about the sternotomy as the access point, you do sternotomies. You also do minimally invasive and even some robotic. How would you categorize the sternotomy versus the other options, if they are options for a patient?

Dr. Mark Berry: For me personally and again, I haven't had any of the surgeries myself but when I think about what needs to be done, I think about what needs to be done on the inside, whether it's heart surgery or lung surgery, whether it's a cancer operation, or whether it's fixing a valve, whether it's bypassing a diseased artery.

For me, what I think about is, what's going to give the best result? If there are a couple options, well, let's do the least risky or the least traumatic. In general, that's how I think about things. If somebody needs heart surgery, there are some surgeries that are just better done as a traditional open sternotomy. That's what I would choose to have if I needed to have that. There are other things, though, that instead of a sternotomy, you may best access from the side, from the right chest. Oftentimes people will call them mini sternotomies. I'm not sure what makes something mini versus maximum. They're all kind of big and they're all kind of traumatic, but in some cases, coming from the side gives a surgeon better visualization of what they need to see. They can do a better job, say, of repairing a valve, than if they were doing the traditional sternotomy. It may be a little bit more complex in some ways but for a specific surgeon that may give them the best access to fix the problem in the best way for the short term and the long term. I would say if a minimally invasive option is considered an option, then I would investigate that. If you can't have a minimally invasive surgery, you're probably still going to do very, very well, but it might be a little bit slower recovery, maybe a little bit more pain, a little bit more time before you're back to completely normal. In six months or a year you're hopefully cured of the cancer, whether the scar was big or small, or your heart is functioning great, whether the incision was big or small. I think if there's an option for minimally invasive surgery, there's not a reason not to do it and it can save people time in the hospital, shorter period of recovery, less pain, medicine, lots and lots and lots of good things and a little bit less risk in a lot of cases. There's less risk of pneumonia or other types of things. If people are investigating options, you're having surgery, those are the things to think about. If somebody tells them I don't think you should have a minimally invasive surgery for this reason, if it sounds like a good reason, then it probably is a good reason.

If it is because, well, I'm personally not comfortable with the minimally invasive surgery, that's also a valid reason. Not all minimally invasive surgery is better than open surgery. If you're interested in a minimally invasive surgery and your surgeon tells you I don't think it's as good in my hands and I prefer to do it as an open, that can be a good reason to go with that surgeon. But it doesn't hurt oftentimes to get another opinion. Maybe see someone who's known to be an expert in a certain technique and see what they say, and then that way, at the very least, people will feel fully informed. They will hopefully not have any regrets later on if things didn't go as well as they hoped. They don't want to look back and say, well, maybe I should have gotten another opinion. I think going in and feeling comfortable with what you've chosen is super important. I try to encourage people to not have remorse afterwards because most people make the best decision they can make with the information they have, with a tough problem, and they're relying on people and oftentimes they make a good decision. Even if things don't turn out perfectly, it doesn't mean it was their fault or that they made a bad decision.

For some people, getting too many opinions can be bad because it can increase the anxiety instead of making you feel better that you're doing the right thing. You may hear something and it sounds a little different, and then it can really throw a lot of confusion. Like wait a minute, even if four people were talking about the same thing, it sounded different and now they're not sure. And then you go for another opinion and then it sounds even more different than the other two and I think that can hurt you. But when it comes time to choose your approach who's going to take care of you, what you're going to have, it's super important to feel comfortable with it. Once you make that decision, I try to tell people you know that's your decision, that's a good decision, you know you made the best decision you could make. Just move forward with it. In most cases it's going to work out very, very well for people.

JH: We see a lot of that on the condition with the unroofing procedure. Now there are robotic options, not for everybody but for some, and then of course, some minimally invasive, depending on the situation. Of course, the sternotomy and the unfortunate part of some people who we've even spoken with you on the podcast, become paralyzed by the analysis, paralysis by analysis, and they can't make a decision and it takes them much longer when, if they would have been able to move quicker, they would have been healed quicker and less symptomatic. So wonderful explanation- and I especially like the fact that you didn't take any sides on it. I was almost going to go leading with the sternotomy is the gold standard, and in fact it really isn't. There are always options.

One thing I didn't have on the question list, Dr. Berry, is you deal in a very high-stress, high-stakes environment on a day-to-day basis and certainly we're appreciative of what you do. What do you do for fun? How does Dr. Berry relax? What hobbies, habits, things do you do that you bring you more joy than what you do for patients?

Dr. Mark Berry: Well, I have a great family, I have a great wife, I have great kids. I am lucky to go home to them. My day always starts and ends great, no matter what happens in between in some way. I like to run, especially being out in California where I live now. It's almost always nice in some way somewhere, whether it's in the early morning or the later afternoon, it's nice to be out. I love music, I love to be an amateur musician, I love to listen to music, and then I like sports and news as well, so I can jump on and read some interesting story about what's going on in the world, or I can read about what's happened with some of the Philadelphia sports teams. Oftentimes, that doesn't bring me joy, but it at least brings me, brings me back to my hometown and back to good memories from when I was growing up.

JH: And what instrument do you play? Is there a particular instrument?

Dr. Mark Berry: I like to play the guitar and then I like playing piano also.

JH: Any final thoughts, anything you want to leave us with?

Dr. Mark Berry: Not really, except I would say for people who are facing some kind of medical procedure, whether it's something like chest surgery or heart surgery or something maybe even more minor, I would just encourage people to be good advocates for themselves and if they find that they're worried about something, they should write it down and they should ask somebody about it. I think that in most cases, they're going to feel better after they get to talk about it and they're going to have, at the very least, a better understanding, and hopefully a more realistic understanding, of whatever it is that they're worried about. Their answer might not always be super comforting but what they're worried about is valid and they should be worried about it. If they can at least talk it over with people, it becomes something that they're actively addressing and I think it takes away some of the fear of just being a passive player. As you're going through whatever medical journey that you need to go through, I think things like you're doing, these podcasts, that are looking at different topics, are a great resource for people. If you've never had heart surgery, you can listen to some people talk about it and, at the very least, you're listening to someone who had heart surgery and they're fine. They sound intelligent. They sound healthy, and that can be important to start with.

DR. JACK BOYD: Let's Cross That Bridge Together

(An explanation of the surgical unroofing procedure.)

In a world where the rhythm of life is mirrored by the beating of our hearts, there exists a cadre of medical artisans who weave themselves into the intricate tapestry of human life—heart surgeons, or more formally, cardiothoracic surgeons.

Among these skilled practitioners is Dr. Jack Boyd, whose name has become synonymous with the procedure known as myocardial bridge "unroofing". His expertise and pioneering spirit are displayed in the interview I was so fortunate to have with him. He most likely has done more "unroofing" procedures than any other doctor in the world and as of the writing of this book had done nearly 250 of these life-saving operations. Here is what he had to say on his first ever podcast experience:

Jeff Holden (Host): Dr Boyd, I can't tell you how excited we are to have you on the program. You are, without doubt, the foremost authority on unroofing surgery in the country, having done more unroofing procedures than any other surgeon doing the procedure. When did you do your first unroofing procedure, and what was it that led you to believe that what you were doing would become such a successful procedure at reducing and, in some cases, eliminating symptoms of a myocardial bridge?

Dr. Jack Boyd (Guest): I first came to Stanford in the fall of 2014. I was coming as a coronary surgeon to do bypass surgeries, all the different types, on-pump and off-pump, and was well-taught on minimally invasive variations of different operations. There was another surgeon here, Scott Mitchell, who had been doing these surgeries and had teamed up with Dr. Ingela Schnittger, who at the time was head of the department researching myocardial bridges. I think they'd been doing them for about three years and done, I don't know 20 or 25 of them. He was moving on when I was coming in and they asked, because it was a natural segue from coronary surgery to this, if I'd be willing to come out a month early to watch him do a couple of procedures. I made an extra trip to Stanford over the summer and watched him do two of them in a single day to see how he did it. That was the end of July, and then I came and joined the group in September. I think October was the first time that I did the surgery. I wanted to make sure that we did them as they'd done them before. It was something unfamiliar to me until I started to develop an experience with it.

JH: I know many of the people reading this are trying to decide on whether the procedure is right for them. What criteria do you consider before surgery becomes valid?

Dr. Jack Boyd: Let me rephrase the way that I think about it just a little from how you asked the question. What we look at is, do we have the appropriate indication for surgery? There is a different way of trying to say the same thing, but in our language it's, do you have the right indication for surgery? The first thing are the symptoms. Generally, there is chest pain with it. There are some symptoms that potentially can be bridge-related like fatigue, weakness, or other things that we can't necessarily directly attribute to bridges, though sometimes we think are associated. Chest pain being the main driving factor.

If there has been nothing else to explain why they've been to the emergency department or to the primary care and onto a cardiologist, has it been demonstrated they haven't had a heart attack, or they don't have reflux? In other words, there isn't another obvious explanation for their chest pain. Frequently, they'd have a stress echo and when it's done here we have some expertise in seeing some objective but very subtle changes in one of the ventricular walls. That can be suggestive and in our program that would probably warrant you medical therapy. We would try a beta blocker to see if that takes care of the symptoms, or a certain calcium channel blocker to see if that helps. If the symptoms persist or the medications don't really cover it, then we look for the anatomic presence of a myocardial bridge and we usually do that with a coronary CT scan and our radiologists can identify the bridges that quantify the length and the depth of the bridge from the CT scan. We start to get more suspicious. The medical management is ongoing. Adjustments are made. It really gets to the point where we say if you have symptoms in a hematologically significant LAD (lateral anterior descending artery) myocardial bridge, that's not tolerable despite maximal medical therapy, then we think surgery could be an option for you.

JH: I'm going to take that one step further now, after the diagnosis, as the most sought after surgeon as a result of your experience and familiarity with the entire process of the unroofing procedure, can you share, for the benefit of those who are just learning the details of the procedure, the steps taken prior to surgery and then exactly what's done once you're in the operating room?

Dr. Jack Boyd: Jeff, I want to recognize one of the points you made. I have this surgical experience because of the team that we have here. Dr. Ingela Schnittger on the echocardiographic and medical side and Dr. Jennifer Tremmel who performs the provocative testing on the interventional cardiology side, our IVUS (intravenous ultrasound) fellows, which rotate every couple years and the chest radiologists who allow us to put this program together and look at so many patients with this medical condition that isn't universally accepted as being a medical condition. Now, skip ahead to when the patient gets in the operating room. They've been through this entire process. They've met with our team, they've been studied, they've met those criteria and when we decide on surgery we always decide the approach prior to surgery.

The two options are a sternotomy, which is what people think of as traditional open-heart surgery through the middle of the chest, or a minimally invasive anterior thoracotomy, a small incision between the ribs in the left chest. The patient goes to the operating room, goes to sleep with anesthesia, we get the breathing tube placed, we put in the appropriate monitoring lines and catheters and then we'll make the incision. To look at the heart when we get there, we position it so we can see where the LAD should be. We can usually see it where it exits the bridge and the distal or the farthest-out aspect. Then we have an instrument, a stabilizer, kind of a U-shaped suction cup that we can place over a part of the heart that holds that portion of the heart still, and that way we can begin the unroofing procedure. Most people's hearts have a little bit of fat on the outside, and so we divide the fat on top. First there are some veins that go through there. We'll control those. We get down to the muscle that overlies the artery, that is the bridge, and then, moving from the farthest point out to the nearest point, we divide the muscle over the top of the artery. Here, we just want to cut in a straight line. Like we learned as children early on.

JH: When you do that, it's an incision of the heart muscle?

Dr. Jack Boyd: When we say incision, we're talking about cutting with a knife, on top. The way I prefer to do this, and this was related to how I was trained to do bypass surgery. I actually take scissors and cut through the muscle like you would a piece of paper.

JH: We don't want to minimize the significance of the procedure, as we're talking about literally cutting of the heart muscle, but fear of the surgery sometimes holds people back from doing what would be in their best interest. Has there ever been a case where a patient did not make it out of the surgery as a result of the procedure?

Dr. Jack Boyd: No. Now, close to 250 of these later, we've had no major complications. My definition of major complications means no death, no stroke, no heart attack, no significant bleeding where they required a re-operation in the short term. This is not to say that there haven't been some minor issues. The most debilitating one is we've seen a few cases of what we call Dressler's syndrome, or an inflammation of the sac around the heart or the sac around the lungs, where you get bad inflammation and pain afterwards or their can be collection of fluid around the heart or the lungs. We've had one or two patients who have required a blood transfusion, received a unit of platelets, and we've also had one or two people who have had some healing problems with the breast bone or the skin above that.

JH: Very low. Very few post-surgical complications for sure.

Dr. Jack Boyd: I think I have trouble completely putting myself in the patient's position, but a lot of the concern of being scared about having cardiac surgery, the risk of major complications-and it's not zero, for us, they've been very low and then I there's the recovery, right? There's a period of time where you're not going to be able to do what you want to do when you want to do it and that's tough to give up that control. I don't want to have to coerce anyone into surgery but I think when the symptoms are so significant and it's the patient driving it, the cost of the surgery is the risk up front and the time to recover. The patients that we've studied, we all think there's a very high likelihood of significant symptomatic improvement. That risk and recovery period are short in the big scheme of things. Hopefully we'll get you back to doing what you were doing before, the way you wanted to do it.

JH: I want to make two comments on that. First, it absolutely is the team and it's the preparation of that team that I can attest to, having gone through the procedure at Stanford. So much takes place on the back end that if that doesn't build confidence, I don't know what does. But the second part is that people are so concerned and what we hear more than anything is the sternotomy part. It's the cutting-open part. That's the hard part and oh boy, is it going to hurt and the pain and well, it's your heart. As they read this, what you're saying gives them some solace, that okay, maybe it's not going to all happen when I want and happen as fast as I want. We're all impatient but, to your point, the body does take time to heal and we need to be concerned about what's important, the condition of the heart.

Dr. Jack Boyd: Yes, and we do offer minimally invasive options as well, so the recovery can be a little bit quicker with that. Sometimes it's actually more painful than the sternotomy and I certainly understand people's reticence to have their chest cracked open. We do this regularly every week, with excellent results, and expect people to be back to 100% within two to three months and really to be 80 or 90% within a month if they have the sternotomy approach, but potentially a little bit quicker the thoracotomy approach. And yes, as the surgeon it's easy for me to downplay the surgical approach because it's not being done to me. But I also want to prioritize the long-term results and not as much on the short-term discomfort.

JH: Agreed. Do you see more incidences in a certain age range than you do in others? Does it tend to be older, younger, middle aged, male, female?

Dr. Jack Boyd: We're still learning a lot about this disease, right? If we go back to that the most basic aspect of it is 20 or 30% of all human beings have an intramyocardial LAD, or what we call a myocardial bridge, at least as far as we can tell, it's only a very small portion that have active symptoms because of that. When we looked at our first 50, 100, and 150, we found that it was usually women, in the 30 to 45 age range. We're in the 250 range now, and I'm only talking about those who progress to surgery.

It's my impression now that we're seeing more men and people up into their 60s and 70s. Also, we're beginning to see some distinctions within the disease itself. So for me, what I call classic, isolated, this being the only problem, is someone without coronary disease associated with the myocardial bridge. They're quite young for someone that's going to go to heart surgery in the 30 to 50 range, and they don't have a fixed blockage from coronary atherosclerosis, but they do have significant symptoms and chest pain when their heart rate gets up and possibly some endothelial dysfunction with it as well. That's one part of the disease. That's just the myocardial bridge plus or minus endothelial dysfunction. We've also looked into this and the flow disturbances that come from the bridge and we do see that all patients have some thickening of the artery before the bridge and we have a question—this is a hypothesis, this isn't known—if that can progress to a certain form of coronary artery disease where there's proximal LAD obstruction from the altered flow dynamics from the bridge that develop farther along in life. It's not necessarily the case. It could also be your cholesterol is way out of whack, you eat McDonald's twice a week, smoke, or something like that, it's a different story. However, if there's actually a mechanical component to the way your heart formed that predisposes you to having significant coronary artery disease, could it be that the bridge is a cause of that?

JH: Dr. Schnittger was very clear in her discussion with us, 100% of the people with a bridge have some semblance of thickening or occlusion where the artery enters the heart.

Dr. Jack Boyd: It's not always occlusion. The tube doesn't always get harder, but the wall always gets thicker and then sometimes, the tube is also getting narrower. Is that because of the bridge or is that because of the more commonly recognized problem of coronary artery disease?

JH: What's your opinion on why this is still seen as such a controversial procedure? What can we do to convince the cardiology community that myocardial bridges are real, they are symptomatic and we've got all these case studies now, hundreds throughout the country, of people who have been improved as a result of the surgery.

Dr. Jack Boyd: As I alluded to earlier, the fact that bridges are so common—we suspect 20 or 30 percent of all people have them—and all of the surgeries that we've done for our patients have been very important in life-changing positively for most, almost all of them. But that's only a small percentage, a fraction of a fraction of a percent of the entire population. So it's very real for the people that have it. How common it is to have a bridge and have it be pathologic or cause symptoms, I think is much, much more rare. That's one thing. Then, medications—whether it be a beta blocker, a calcium channel blocker, nitrate-based medication, those are generally seen as pretty reasonable—but surgery for something like this seems quite radical, right? We have done lots of planning and have very good results for our patients, but it still is heart surgery. There is a risk that a coronary artery can be damaged. Sometimes the coronary artery runs through the ventricle. It's not without risk and at some point there likely will be a major complication. Humans have had myocardial bridges for the entirety of history, and we haven't conclusively demonstrated that it causes sudden cardiac death. I understand how people are slow to accept in the medical community, and that establishment of the community is slow to accept it as a real problem. I think, more than convincing, it's really developing a good relationship with your physicians so that you can have a conversation. When I first heard about it in 2014, I thought, maybe I heard about this in medical school, but we certainly didn't pay any attention to it. I look at it more as developing good patient-physician relationships, being able to have a conversation about it.

Our program is really continuing to do quite a bit of research into it. What group of people is it most commonly found in? What are the hemodynamic factors that predispose one to having symptoms? What is their natural history? Can this be a life-threatening condition? *Is* this a life-threatening condition? Is there another medicine that could treat the symptoms that people could avoid having heart surgery? I think those are some of the reasons.

And then we have still yet to collect beyond-symptom surveys, a significant amount of objective data, or that hemodynamic data after the surgery to show that the surgery has changed something physiologically and be able to make that connection from the bridge and its squeeze, to the symptoms that you experience. Did those measurements change after the surgery? How much of this has a placebo component? We don't know if the bridge is a risk for sudden cardiac death. We have seen some minor heart attacks from isolated bridges, how it may play a role in the development of coronary artery disease. All those things together can contribute to why it's not universally accepted as a disease.

JH: Do you think the information that's being conveyed today is effective in getting more and more cardiologists to understand, and at least appreciate, the reality of the symptoms?

Dr. Jack Boyd: Yes. I would say in the first five years that I was doing this, when patients would come and travel to us, the story we received was, the physician that they were working with was not on board with them. Your podcast, how many listeners you've had, and certainly the Facebook group and the literature that our group has published, are bringing it to awareness. Our surgical societies are also starting to mention it. It's gaining critical mass, it's becoming so that people are more aware of it, and that's certainly the intent here.

JH: Many people are considering the surgery, they're apprehensive about the sternotomy and they're hearing about robotic surgical unroofing at this point- and obviously, it's less pain, faster recovery times, less trauma to the body. Can you comment a little bit about what you're seeing in terms of robotic unroofing at this point?

Dr. Jack Boyd: One of the main limitations for robotic surgery is that the main surgical robot no longer maintains the appropriate equipment for the current edition of the surgical robot to do the surgery. I know it's been done and been done safely. I'm not sure it's going to be universally applicable because there are situations that may require a different approach as a result of the particular placement of the bridged segment of the artery and I see that as being potentially problematic.

With the robotic approach, I certainly recognize its appeal. Having your chest cracked open is worse than having a minimally invasive surgery is worse than having a robotic surgery from the patient's perspective. So certainly, with minimally invasive, if you can perform the same surgery and do it with less trauma, that's a better thing. I agree with that completely. I do minimally invasive valve surgeries. I do robotically assisted bypass surgeries. I think that's the way we should be headed. The equipment doesn't exist to do it for everyone at this time and there are going to be some people that aren't going to be candidates based on their anatomy.

The perception that it's a quick fix and that you're going to have it one day and go back and be completely normal tomorrow is unrealistic at this time.

JH: I do think many people see it as the panacea to the challenges of everything else, right? A lot of people are just waiting, and in some cases they're wasting quality of life time, whereas a healing of eight to 12 weeks from a sternotomy really is relatively short when you think about it in the grand scheme of things.

Dr. Jack Boyd: Yes, I can understand how. I'm not the one going through that. It's a balance of what the symptoms are and how difficult that is for you on a day-to-day basis and what your own internal value system is, from what costs you're willing to pay to have a very good chance of having those symptoms go away.

JH: I'm going to shift a little bit on you. Yours is truly a career of life and death. In so many cases, that, to me, is incomprehensible in terms of the stress. What is it you do to unwind? What does somebody like Dr. Jack Boyd, who's in people's hearts and chests all day long, do to relax and have fun? I know you do take vacations, because I had to wait a week for my surgery while you came back from one. But what is it that you do, Dr. Boyd? How do you relax?

Dr. Jack Boyd: Well, Jeff, I have a wonderful wife and four terrific children, so a lot of my time away from work is doing fun things with them or driving them around to extracurricular activities. We do like to take time off when the kids are out of school to go visit family or go see somewhere that we haven't been before. Since relocating to California, I've developed an interest in surfing so I'm learning how to surf and generally like hiking, biking, reading books, the things that I think most people enjoy doing.

JH: The values that California brings to us in terms of its topography, its geography, everything else make it great for all those things.

Dr. Jack Boyd: There's so much available to do here pretty much any day of the year.

JH: If there was one thing we could leave everyone with, knowing the majority of the people who are paying attention to the podcast have a myocardial bridge, is there a suggestion that you could give as the best thing you can do for yourself? Obviously, it's individual, but if you could say something to the effect of Jeff, here's the one thing I'd like you to consider as you consider the options of how to deal with this bridge. What might that look like?

Dr. Jack Boyd: I think of it as being their own self-advocate in recognizing the medical team that they form around them or form with them to work through this problem is on their side. Someone outside of our program may not have a lot of experience or exposure with myocardial bridges, but they're in their profession generally because they want to help people. It can be difficult if a patient presents with symptoms and the doctor or nurse practitioner doesn't have the fix for them, I would say hang in there, keep your head up, continue to work through it, and certainly by all means contact us in our program to help work through this. There's literature available that we can present in the right manner to the people that they're working with to help them gain some understanding and know that if their problems are because of a myocardial bridge, there is a potential solution for them that can make them feel a lot better.

JH: Self-advocacy is so important, as we know. Just because you get told one time it's anxiety, it's stress, whatever, which we know happens quite often, you have to keep going and you have to keep asking the questions and if you really believe and you really feel and you know your body, then that condition is real. There's an answer out there someplace.

Dr. Jack Boyd: You know your body better than *we* do. You have to give us some time to catch up and figure it out.

JH: I think *you* know mine better than I do, at least inside! I've been blessed to have been introduced to you as a result of my condition, Dr. Boyd, and I have the utmost appreciation for what you do. I'm eternally grateful for the fact that you are my surgeon, as most people know, and I've been asymptomatic since the surgery, what a blessing that is. Your surgical skill allowed me to return to the physical condition I was in a couple of years ago.

I remember the day that I was leaving the hospital. You showed up and it was a Saturday when you could have been spending time with your family or hiking or learning to surf. You were very casual, which was really nice to see, and we had a conversation in the hallway and I said you know what, I do podcasts for a living, I'm going to do a podcast about this and I would love to have you on. And here we are. So I thank you for that. I thank you for your time, for sharing your experience and for giving so many people the hope and knowing that there are solutions to relieving the symptoms of these crazy myocardial bridges. It's my opinion that the world's a better place because of what you are doing and what your team at Stanford is doing, and I cannot thank you enough. I thank you from the very, very bottom of my imperfect heart.

Dr. Jack Boyd: Thank you, Jeff.

DR. HUSAM BALKHY:
Bring in the Bots

(Unroofing the myocardial bridge robotically.)

The nexus where technology meets medicine has revolutionized the field of cardiac care. I had the privilege of discussing this innovation with Dr. Husam Balkhy, a trailblazer in the realm of cardiac surgery. Dr. Balkhy's journey is a testament to the power of innovation, the importance of adaptability, and the endless quest for improved patient outcomes.

Dr. Husam Balkhy is professor of surgery and director of robotic and minimally invasive cardiac surgery at the University of Chicago Medicine. He received his cardiothoracic and vascular surgery training at Tufts New England Medical Center and Lehigh Clinic in Boston, Massachusetts. He was chair of cardiac surgery at the Wisconsin Heart Hospital in Milwaukee, Wisconsin, prior to moving to the University of Chicago in July 2013. Dr. Balkhy is considered a pioneer of robotic cardiac surgery, having performed over 2,000 cases by mid-2022. He has the largest series of robotic, totally endoscopic coronary bypass operations in the world, with over 1,000 cases. He is a frequently sought after speaker and proctor worldwide and has trained multiple surgeons, both nationally and internationally, in robotic cardiac surgical techniques.

Jeff Holden (Host): Dr. Balkhy, can you give us a little bit of the background on what brought you to robotic surgery versus traditional sternotomy? You started out as a classically trained surgeon, isn't that correct?

Dr. Husam Balkhy (Guest): Yes, that is true. I went through the traditional cardiac surgical training pathway that requires one to be proficient in traditional techniques and open-heart surgery. That was back in the 1990s. I finished my first general surgery training program which was five years, six years because I did some research and then did a vascular surgery fellowship to learn how to operate on blood vessels. I then did my cardiac surgery fellowship, all on the East Coast in Boston, and came out an enthusiastic young heart surgeon ready to go and learned how to do all the techniques with opening people's chest. It became very quickly apparent to me that the invasiveness of what I was doing was significant. Even though we did a great job on the heart, patients would sometimes have lots of trouble with the sawing open of the breastbone. I quickly decided that there were some operations for which I really didn't need to saw people's chests open to get an efficacious result. I started about three years after my beginning practice. I was in Milwaukee at the time and I started trying to minimize the invasiveness of my techniques. The first thing that I did was I eliminated cardiopulmonary bypass when I did somebody's coronary bypass surgery. Cardiopulmonary bypass is a heart-lung machine and stopping of the heart and things like that. I decided that this is an epicardial operation, meaning it's on the surface of the heart and it does not require the heart to be stopped. What I did was, even with sternotomy and with opening the chest, I said, okay, we don't need to really do this. Then, a year or two later, I started working on patients who had atrial fibrillation and approaching their cardiac surgery through little holes using thoracoscopy. That was a new technique that was evolving at the time, in the early 2000s. It allowed me to observe the heart from the side as opposed to from the front. That's one of the major things that I tell junior folks these days, when they're learning to do these less invasive approaches, is to familiarize yourself with what the heart looks like from the side, whether it's the left side or the right side.

Eventually, I moved on to doing less invasive valve surgery. Finally, in 2006, I found a robot and that was the epitome of less invasive heart surgery. I adopted my technique of off-pump coronary bypass through a sternotomy, which is otherwise known as OPCAB, to off-pump coronary bypass using a robot with no chest opening, just little holes. That's called T-CAB. I started doing T-CAB in 2006 and I now have the largest series of T-CAB patients in the world and have been doing it for all those years successfully.

In the process of doing T-Cab there were coronary arteries that were not accessible on the surface of the heart. If you look at the veins on the back of your hand and you can see the veins, that's where a coronary usually lives, on the surface of the heart. There are some coronaries that can be deep and covered by fat, but they can also be deep covered by muscle. In the process of doing T-Cab we were approaching all different types of anatomies and I was digging coronaries out under the muscle to do bypass surgery. These were not people with bridges or anything of that nature or symptomatic bridges, I should say. These were people who just had a deep coronary artery that we were going after to bypass and we're doing that robotically, with little holes, without a sternotomy, without a heart-lung machine, and that was way back in 2008, 2009. These cases are not that frequent, but as you increase your experience you can do them successfully and safely.

In 2010, when I was still in Milwaukee, one of my cardiologists presented a patient who had a myocardial bridge and had worked that patient up aggressively. The reason I say that is because myocardial bridge is not an uncommon condition that cardiologists see on their angiograms. That patient was worked up aggressively and the cardiologist came to the conclusion that this is a significant and clinically relevant myocardial bridge- and I said well, you know, we've been digging coronaries out with the robot. Why don't we do this case? There's no bypass involved. We can go in and it's actually going to be easier for me because I don't have to bypass anything. I can just dig out the coronary and it'll be great.

JH: If you're digging out coronaries from heart muscle tissue and fat, is this different from what would be considered a myocardial bridge unroofing?

Dr. Husam Balkhy: Not different at all. It's just the effect of the coronary being under the muscle that would be different, and how tight the muscle constricts it, how thick the muscle band is. The act of dividing the muscle on top of the coronary is exactly the same. The techniques, the precautions, the measures that we take when we do it one way or the other, it's exactly the same, and so to me it was a no-brainer.

The challenge then became which patients do you actually take to do that too? It's still invasive, it's anesthesia, it's heart surgery, and there are a lot of patients with bridges, and so the challenge wasn't necessarily can you do it. The challenge was whom do you do it to? We began doing that in 2009. I moved to Chicago, University of Chicago in 2013, and in that 10-year period, now it's 2023, we've done about 40 patients.

We haven't done a lot. One of the reasons is that we're very, very selective about who we think benefits from this operation, from unroofing in general, not just robotic unroofing, who benefits from unroofing. We've evolved a very kind of meticulous, if you will, and geographic testing in the cath lab with one of my colleagues, Dr. John Blair, and he was interrogating these bridges very, very closely and we would collaborate and combine to figure out who would benefit, who actually is symptomatic from their bridge because, as noted, a bridge is not uncommon. If we had a cath right now, maybe one of us has a bridge, and if you do have a bridge, you can have it unroofed. So, yes, so you come from the perspective of, well, yeah, and so it's not an uncommon thing. I'm always, first, do no harm. We're not doctors who treat with pills, and when we cut somebody, we take it really, really seriously that we're cutting for the right reason. Even though this is a less invasive operation, we like to get our indications down pat.

JH: The consensus from both people that I'm aware of who've had robotic surgery, as well as those who are contemplating the next step is boy, the sternotomy is tough. As you have said and I know from experience, it's very invasive and it takes a long time to heal. The benefits that so many see with the robotic approach is the healing time, back-to-work sooner, less pain, and I know a lot of people are very, very concerned about both the pain and the visual look. Can you speak to what that looks like in the actual process of robotic surgery? What happens in the post-surgery healing?

Dr. Husam Balkhy: During the surgery itself, we insert little ports, the size of which are about 8 to 10 millimeters in diameter, so slightly larger than a Bic pen. Take out the Bic pen, take out the innards of it and then you have now a hollow tube. That hollow tube is placed through the ribs very carefully. We then insert through those tubes those "ports" we call them, a camera that has 3D magnification, 3d imaging and 10 times magnification with a very high quality picture, as well as wristed robotic instruments, and we work through that.

In the case of a myocardial bridge, it probably takes about anywhere from two to four hours to unroof somebody's bridge. We put a chest tube in at the end through one of the holes, and the chest tube is about the size of one of those 10 millimeter holes and that chest tube stays in overnight. They go to the recovery room, but in our hospital we do it in the ICU. They usually get extubated, meaning the breathing tube comes out at the time of surgery in the operating room, so they don't wake up with a tube in between their vocal cords, which is extremely irritating and not fun. Then they're in pain for about 24 hours until that tube comes out.

The majority of the patients will go home on the day after surgery or the day after that and a majority of our patients don't even unseal the prescription that we give them for narcotic pain medicine because their pain is really controllable with Advil or Ibuprofen or whatnot. The majority are back to full activity within two to three weeks. Definitely a job, but even some are back to exercise and those kinds of things. There are no restrictions after the surgery in terms of lifting and physical activity. I tell them to do whatever they feel like, as long as they're not sore. There is some soreness in the left chest, obviously from the holes that we made.

JH: I know some people who have had robotic surgery who, the second day out, were out and walking around town and actually felt good. To your point, no narcotics. I think Tylenol is what one of the gentlemen was using. He said it's just amazing. In the process you had mentioned something about so many of us having a myocardial bridge and I think the estimate is maybe as many as a third of the population could have a bridge. It's a much smaller percentage that are symptomatic. Is there anything that you particularly look for that says, okay, this is likely a surgical procedure that will benefit this individual, versus trying the medical process or the fact that maybe the bridge isn't even the root cause of their problem?

Dr. Husam Balkhy: Yes, good question. In all honesty, I have had patients that came back positive from the angiographic stress testing that we do in the cath lab and I've still felt reluctant about doing surgery on them and that's because their symptoms just didn't fall into what I would consider something that could be explained by poor blood supply to the heart muscle. What we're talking about here is a constriction that happens in the blood flow of the main coronary artery that feeds the heart muscle, and that constriction happens every time the heart squeezes. On first encounter, that is an oxymoron, because we know that blood flow to the heart muscle occurs not when the heart is *squeezing*, it occurs when the heart is *relaxing*. Who cares what's happening when the heart is squeezing in terms of blood flow to the muscle? That's not when the muscle gets its nourishment. It gets its nourishment when the heart's relaxed.

Many surgeons and cardiologists will say to you that unroofing myocardial bridges is a phantom operation. The way we get beyond it is by testing in the cath lab and demonstrating that when a patient is stressed, the heart is working overtime and beating fast and hard, simulating an exercise or simulating a stressful situation. That squeeze lasts into the phase of diastole, which is the phase of relaxation to some extent, and actually contributes to poor blood supply during the phase when the heart needs to be supplied. Those of us who've done these operations and have seen the patients and have talked to them and listened to what they say are believers in the fact that this works.

Not every heart surgeon will agree with that because of the prevalence of myocardial bridges that are asymptomatic in the community: Why are some symptomatic and some not? The other question is why would some people become symptomatic at a later age in life? This didn't happen as an acquired thing. You're born with the course of your arteries and maybe you could say, well, the heart muscle gets thicker and stronger over time and that's why this evolves.

There's also this notion of endothelial change (referring to the single layer of cells which line the inside of blood vessels, lymph vessels and the heart). These are things that are a little bit beyond my understanding. I'm just what I call the "cutting" doctor. The smart cardiologist understands endothelial disease much better and a lot of patients are treated with medications to help with spasms. There are different things going on in this process that we don't understand yet, and I think patient selection, like I had mentioned earlier, is really the challenge as to whom do you subject to this type of an intervention? We try to minimize the number of people who are not going to benefit from it, because what you've done is you've just subjected them to an operation for which they could have complications and no benefit. Unnecessary.

JH: If you have vasospasms, endothelial dysfunction, your artery is also spasming, the heart spasms and in some cases that constriction of blood flow could be through the whole process, the squeeze, the vasospasm, and then your heart does get starved, which is what it was in my case. And to your point of somebody having a condition asymptomatically, one of the questions that just keeps going through my mind is if so many people have the condition, the myocardial bridge, they appear asymptomatic. But is it possible that they're asymptomatic until they aren't and it's once and this symptom occurs and it's sudden cardiac arrest and that's it? We'll never know, because we don't do autopsies on everybody who passes from what looks like a coronary occlusion or blockage of some sort.

Dr. Husam Balkhy: That's interesting. I don't think there's anything that's been described that this condition can cause sudden cardiac arrest. Otherwise, you'd see a lot more people getting intervention for it. This is what we call a dynamic obstruction, because it's not always there. For example, when the coronary artery comes off the aorta in an abnormal position and it's positioned between the two main blood vessels, the aorta and the pulmonary artery, when we exercise, those blood vessels get more dilated. If you imagine that the two arteries are like this, there's a coronary artery in between them, and when you exercise, they get a little bit bigger and they can pinch the coronary artery. When you are done exercising and things go back to normal, then the pass is fine. That's the dynamic obstruction. That condition has been known to cause sudden death. When somebody's diagnosed with that anomalous coronary artery between the major vessels, that's an indication for surgery. We do bypass or unroofing or things of that nature to rectify that problem.

JH: You're going in with a very small tool, robotically. What happens to the chest cavity? How do you get enough room to work on top of the heart when you're in there robotically, versus opening somebody up?

Dr. Husam Balkhy: Great question and this is what I want to talk about directly to your community. First thing we do is begin to insufflate carbon dioxide inside the chest in order to create the space. Normally our chest cavities are occupied by the organs, two lungs and a heart, and then all the mediastinal fat and things like that surround it that completely occupy the space. For us to get to the heart, we've got to collapse the left lung and that's easily done. It's not a permanent condition and it can be uncollapsed very quickly at the drop of a hat. Nobody needs to worry about the fact that we're collapsing their left lung. When you go on a heart lung machine for regular open heart surgery, you're collapsing both lungs.

I always get that question oh, you collapsed my lung, how's that going to go? Am I going to be okay? And the answer is yes, you're going to be okay, because it's a natural thing. We collapse the lung and that gives us the space. Now imagine your chest with no lung occupying it. That's all the space we need.

The thing that facilitates this operation endoscopically using a robotic approach is something called an endo wrist stabilizer and it's an instrument on a version of the robot that is called the S I. That S I has been around now for about 15 or so years and it's being replaced by the newer system, which came out in 2014 or 2015, called the X I. The robot that I use for any coronary intervention, whether it's coronary bypass or myocardial bridge or several other operations on the surface of the heart, I use the old system which we still have at our hospital. Many surgeons don't have that old system anymore. When I say old I don't mean it's old and outdated. It's a great system. It's actually, in my mind, better than the newer system. I use the newer system for other types of robotic heart surgeries.

But the message that I want to relay is that this system and stabilizer are not available for the newer generations of robot, and my ability to do this operation will cease to exist once we phase out completely this S I robot, which will happen probably in about a year and a half. Because surgeons have not adopted this approach, whether it's for coronary bypass or for the other procedures, of which one is bridge unroofing, the company hasn't felt the need to make a stabilizer that can assist us in doing this operation totally endoscopically with the newer robot, or the X I version.

Because the myocardial bridge community is very active, which I've noticed, I think that they can be a voice or you can be a voice in helping the industry understand that some of these instruments are vital to these operations and they need to be. They need to continue to provide them to those of us who are interested. It may not be a huge amount of volume that they're going to get out of this type of an instrument, it's not like prostate surgery that is done robotically but it is a vital piece of what we do on the heart that when it goes away, I won't be able to do this operation anymore.

JH: We have enough challenges getting cardiologists to accept the fact that our symptoms are real. We certainly don't need those who accept that they are real that are helping us, to be challenged. That's just another consequence we don't need to have at this point.

You mentioned in one of the videos that I saw on the University of Chicago website, haptic feedback, which is something that you don't get from the mechanics of the robot at this point. If you were surgically in there with your hands, you could feel the density of the tissue as you were cutting and you would understand a little bit more by feel. How has that challenged you or how have you accommodated the situation where you don't have that sense of feel that you don't get from the robot?

Dr. Husam Balkhy: It's a matter of experience and learning curve. When you first start operating with these tools, you have no clue how much pressure you're exerting on the tissue. The cases will take longer, because you're still trying to develop your sense of dimensions and tension and pressure and things like that. As you get more and more experienced, you develop what is sometimes called visual haptic feedback, for example, when I use a very, very fine suture and I want to tie it, I can't really feel the tension that I'm exerting on the stitch or the thread, so what I end up doing is using my visualization to understand different cues. That, generally, will give me the feedback that I need.

If I, for example, want to see how hard or stiff a coronary artery is and whether it's calcified or not, I move it around and kind of see how it responds. So, even though I can't really feel the softness or the hardness of the vessel, I know how hard it is by just having done it hundreds of times. Visual haptic feedback is a thing and that's why we rely on it to help us.

Would it be nice to have a haptic feedback system? Absolutely. There are some robot companies that are working on that, but it's not there yet.

JH: I figure if they can get the steering wheel in a car to tell you when you're crossing over the lane by vibration, I'm sure they're going to get there. With AI now and technology for the robot, what are some of the concerns? Post robotic surgery may be different than traditional sternotomy recovery, correct?

Dr. Husam Balkhy: Yes, good question. There are a couple of concerns but they're minor. One of them is the fact that we use carbon dioxide to insufflate the chest and create the space, that can be sometimes caustic on the tissues. We treat that with medication for four or five days after surgery. Sometimes it's a course of steroids, sometimes it's other medications and anti-inflammatory medicine.

JH: Of the 40 patients that you've done so far for bridge repair, how many of them have said they experienced significant improvements in their capabilities or significant decreases in their pain or symptoms?

Dr. Husam Balkhy: 82.9% wonderful, and I would imagine the other 17% have probably got some co-morbidities or other issues that are plaguing them. And that's, I think, as we're getting more experienced and we're learning, a function of better selecting the patients. Patient selection is a word that you hear a lot in the medical literature and people who present their results, to me, I would love to say to you, 99% of our patients have excellent improvement in their pain-but what it means is that I've excluded a lot of patients to get to that number. In this case I've included 17% who may or may not have had a positive result and unfortunately, they didn't, but we may have, in that process of decreasing our threshold, included another 15% who did.

There's this notion in general surgery that you have to have a certain percentage of what they call negative laparotomies (a major surgical procedure that involves making a large incision in the abdomen to examine its organs). This is in the treatment of appendicitis, which we know is a terrible disease but it's a very easy fix. You get your appendix taken out If you have it inflamed, and so there are some patients who come in with belly pain, middle of the night, you just can't be sure. So you got taken to the ER and you take them to the OR and you find that you have what they call a negative lap, meaning the appendix is perfectly fine and it's not inflamed and you didn't have to take them to the OR.

When we're really, really selective, and I am *very* selective, as I mentioned before, we'd have a success rate of 99%, but we don't, and I think it's okay and we do see people who have gone through the opportunity of submission to surgeons who are doing robotic surgery and get declined.

JH: Clearly there are other issues that the surgeon is looking at, saying it just isn't going to work for you and I think that's the best thing you can do, because to have that false expectation of improvement is worse than understanding that you have some complications that may require a sternotomy or you may have other situations where you may not even be a candidate for the unroofing procedure.

Dr. Husam Balkhy: Well, I want to explain. One thing is that when people get denied robotic myocardial bridge unroofing in my practice, it's not because there are technical difficulties or that it cannot be done robotically, I can do it with a sternotomy. That is not the reason that they get declined. The reason they get declined is because we don't think that they would benefit from an unroofing procedure because of their symptoms being not perfectly aligned with what this disease does or because their angiographic interrogation, what we call provocative testing, is not positive from the technical aspect. There is not a myocardial bridge that we can't handle robotically. It's not like we need to do a sternotomy because of this or that or the other. When you're experienced at robotic surgery, you can handle the majority of bridges, all of them. Indeed, the robotic approach sometimes allows you to do a more extensive, myocardial bridge unroofing than a non-robotic approach.

JH: So the depth, the length, the possible multiple bridges really are not of any significance in robotic.

Dr. Husam Balkhy: Nope, endoscopic. When we do a robotic bypass, there are two types of robotic bypass. One is where the whole procedure is done with the robot, we need that stabilizer, and we harvest the conduit from the chest wall, called the internal mammary artery. We bypass endoscopically using the robotic instruments. The second variety, which is actually the more common, unfortunate because of the lack of the stabilizer and the utilization of it, is where the robot is used to harvest the conduit and then the surgeon makes a small incision between your fourth and fifth rib and goes in and does the surgery to bypass with the hands, with the regular suture technique. And the reason that this can be limiting is because now you are limited in looking at the LAD through a small five to seven centimeter incision with a little bit of rib spreading, and all you have is one area where you can work on and you can't go distally, you can't go proximally, you can't go to another area whereas with the endoscopic approach, imagine having this 10 times magnification scope with this 3D vision inside in between the fourth and fifth rib or the third and fourth rib, and you can move that scope all up and down the chest and get to any part of what is inside the chest and deal with it.

If you've got a bridge up top and you've got a bridge down bottom, you can take care of both of them using that approach. What I liken it to is if you're at the Louvre and you want to see the Mona Lisa and all they gave you was a little hole in the wall to be able to find the right angle to see that beautiful smile, well, you're going to have to really work hard to see it and you may not even be able to see it. But if they gave you a high definition magnified scope and put it in through even a smaller hole, you can direct that scope wherever you want. You can magnify, you can bring it in, you can actually move it in, you can take it out and you can see the Mona Lisa significantly better.

JH: It's that zoom on our phones that we all use to see something closer. Now let's shift gears just a little bit. What do you do to relax? What's a little bit of downtime for Dr. Balkhy when he's not literally saving lives?

Dr. Husam Balkhy: Oh, downtime, I would say I cycle. That's good to do. I love listening to podcasts, which is a thing that everybody does these days. It's an interesting kind of revolution, if you will. I like to ski. I play some tennis. I've played much more in the past, but those are the kinds of things that I'll do if I have some time.

JH: Could you tell me what the best process is for anybody interested to go through to reach out to you?

Dr. Husam Balkhy: I think the best way to get a direct interaction, as opposed to sending an email or going on the website or anything like that, is to call my office. I have a wonderful robotic coordinator. Her name is Ruth Buckner and I have a wonderful team. My nurse practitioners and my physician assistants, we're all marshaled towards what I call the robotic revolution. Whether it's in myocardial bridge or coronary surgery or valve surgery or arrhythmia surgery, all of that can be done in our practice using the robot, and the number to call is 773-834-1612. I've seen enough patients to convince me, and the fact that we have at our fingertips a totally less invasive procedure for which the risk is very low and the encumbrance to recovery is also quite limited, robotic is a revelation and we should take advantage of it.

If I had a patient who was equivocal in the indications for surgery and all I had was a saw and a heart lung machine, I don't think I would subject that person to that. But if I can do it stealth, with four little holes and a chest tube and they go home in a day or two, that might be the way to get to a larger number of people that you could say well, if it was the bridge, thankfully the symptoms are gone and that the problem has been treated. If it wasn't the bridge, then the encumbrance was not that severe and the risk to you and to your health was not that significant. And you've got four little mosquito bites to show for it, then we'll go find what the problem really was.

To see the complete robotic unroofing procedure I was fortunate enough to attend, visit the "Imperfect Heart" YouTube channel and search "Cutting the Heart: Robotic Unroofing of a Myocardial Bridge with Dr. Husam Balkhy."

THE INTERVIEWS

Edited Transcripts From "Imperfect Heart" Podcast Episodes

THE PATIENTS

DR. LINDA CUNNINGHAM: They Didn't Teach This In Med School

(A doctor's effort to get to surgery.)

Many of you have not yet had surgery. Many of you may not even have had complete diagnosis as to the severity of your condition other than to be in various degrees of discomfort or pain, and depending on that severity, concern for your very own lives. I get it. Uncertainty of our condition is one of the worst places to be.

I have had many inquiries from listeners to the Imperfect Heart episodes, each one as unique as the other, each one as moving. For me, these are quite emotional as I understand where many of my listeners are coming from. What I've seen, in addition to those incredible stories of perseverance and pursuit to accomplish the goal of proper diagnosis to relief of symptoms through the most appropriate means is that many of you are still in the process stage. Still wondering what's wrong. Still waiting for formal tests to determine if surgery is an option, a relief from the symptoms our bridges create. Interviews that I do with those not yet post-surgery are called "Journeys" as you'll hear from the next two people. "Journeys" is meant to be everything up to the surgery that may help others in the same space. Those looking for answers, debunking myths, and taking their health into their own process of advocacy.

Imagine being a retired internal medicine physician, having run countless marathons, climbed mountains and enjoyed an active lifestyle, only to be confronted by an unfamiliar heart condition. That's precisely the conundrum Dr. Linda Cunningham faced. Despite being a medical professional herself, she was initially taken aback by her diagnosis of myocardial bridging. Her active lifestyle had always been a testament to her health, but as she discovered, even the fittest armor is susceptible to hidden battles.

Dr. Cunningham is a 66-year-old retired, board-certified internal medicine physician with the same condition with so many similar attributes that we've all come to know when you have a myocardial bridge. She's a native of Illinois, graduate of University of Illinois College of Medicine, and is now retired in Salem, Oregon after practicing there for 21 years. She's a mother of three adult children, and has been married to her husband, Ed, also a doctor, for 42 years.

Jeff Holden (Host): You were just settling in to enjoy the fruits of your labor and then this happens.

Dr. Linda Cunningham (Guest): I had actually retired in 2015, so I had settled into retirement. But yes, this diagnosis and my increasing symptoms put a huge damper on my physical activities.

JH: It's interesting because we've had other guests on the program and everybody's situation is different in terms of the way the symptoms appear. Some are over a long period of time that they've known something was wrong and they were getting the improper diagnosis because nobody was thinking heart.

Dr. Linda Cunningham: Right.

JH: And then others like you or I, where all of a sudden, everything was good and then it wasn't so well.

Dr. Linda Cunningham: Actually, it wasn't for me. I was astounded when I looked back through my medical records. I saved things from visits and all. I had actually been complaining of chest pain on and off since 2006 and I had just completely pushed it out of my mind. I looked back though.

I had had an echocardiogram. I had physician visits, I had ER visits. I totally ignored them or felt that because nothing was found on those tests, and because I had been a marathon runner or was still a marathon runner, it couldn't possibly be my heart.

JH: There's a word for that.

Dr. Linda Cunningham: Denial. The subtitle of my life is Denial Runs Deep.

JH: So tell us a little bit about your love of sport, the things that you've been doing that you no longer can do at this point, how experienced you were and how active you were prior to the symptoms.

Dr. Linda Cunningham: I had always been an active person. We loved to hike, backpack, snowshoe, downhill ski, kayak. I had been a marathon runner, a Triathlete. We had taken long distance bike rides. You, name it. I'd done it. We climbed a mountain here in Oregon.

I pushed myself and I enjoyed pushing myself. It felt good in my marathons. I was, I wouldn't say competitive, I didn't qualify for Boston, but I came very close. I really wanted to push my body to see how far I could go. One of the times that led to an emergency room visit was after a long run of about 20 miles training for a marathon. I decided on the hill coming back up to our house I'd push myself. That didn't work out. I had chest pain. Ended up going to the emergency room, and of course they found nothing, even though they did the usual cardiac enzyme testing. I got sent home, but then it was a few years later when I had chest pain that kind of came on and off with lesser exercise that I finally went in and said something has to be done.

I was admitted, this was about 2017. I was headed to the ICU and I had an angiogram done, and the doctor who did my angiogram said, good news, your coronary arteries look beautiful, wide open. Nothing wrong except you have this little bridge, but lots of people have that, and it's nothing to worry about. Just keep your heart rate low. I was about to take off on the Camino Del Santiago, which is a hiking pilgrimage across northern Spain. And we ended up hiking 400 miles in 40 days over the Pyrenees and several other mountain ranges. I got chest pain and I vividly remember going into a pharmacy in Pamplona, Spain and picking up Zantac because I thought, oh, I'm getting GERD (acid reflux). It was the bridge giving me problems.

JH: Yes. Not knowing, that's going to be the cause when we experience the chest pain. In my case, it would be the vasospasms that would create ventricular tachycardia.

As it got worse, almost every time, if I had a severe vasospasm episode, I would go into VT (ventricular tachycardia, a condition in which the lower chambers of the heart beats too quickly). Not good.

Dr. Linda Cunningham: Back in 2017, when the doctor said I had this problem, he said, just keep your heart rate low, but you really don't need medications. He did prescribe me metoprolol, but I didn't want to take medicine and I was doing pretty well. So we continued to hike, although there were a few times when we were hiking more recently in the past couple of years when going up a steep hill, it bothered me.

I just said, well, I'll back off a little bit and it'll be okay. Early January, we did a hike that we had done before, but going up a hill, I experienced the pain and even coming down the hill, it was still there and I said, oh, this isn't good. A few days later we went snowshoeing at about 4,000-foot elevation, and I had it pretty much the whole snowshoe trip. I said I need to check this out. And that's when I went back to the cardiologist and started having testing, including a routine treadmill test with the EKG apparatus. And it was very positive. I could see that myself. I was having some chest pain during the exam, but I still pushed myself because I wanted to get a good test, right? The cardiologist later came in and looked at it and said, "I think this is a false positive" even though he was looking at S T depressions with down-sloping that I had seen umpteen times in my career. And he was still calling it a false positive. I trusted this man. He was the one who had done my angiogram, but I don't think that was good advice. I had an adenosine test, but my heart rate didn't get high enough to give an adequate test. My heart rate was 64. We took off for a trip to Hawaii. I get the call in Hawaii. Oh, your adenosine test was negative. Which is great. It didn't show any ischemia (reduced blood flow), but that's not really proof one way or another whether my chest pain was due to the bridge. I did a lot of slow beach walks in Hawaii and just waited it out and then got put on medicine and slowed way, way down to try to prevent chest pain from coming on.

JH: Has the chest pain become more and more frequent over the course of this last year now?

Dr. Linda Cunningham: Yes, very much so. Since January it suddenly got a lot worse. Until January, my husband and I routinely would walk seven, sometimes 10 miles at a time. And I was having no problems. We weren't speed walking, but we were going maybe three to three-and-a-half miles an hour. Which is a pretty good clip. Now I'm walking about one mile an hour because if I go any faster, I get breathless or get chest pain. Instead of zipping around my neighborhood, walking fast, walking long distances, walking with my group of friends who walk fairly briskly, now I am at my snail's pace around the block. And not comfortable. It doesn't feel like me.

JH: I hear so many other people with the same situation who don't have a clue what's going on. They're not even aware that it's something with their heart yet until they figure it out and somebody does give them a proper diagnosis. In our correspondence, you actually mentioned that you've never even heard of a myocardial bridge when you were practicing, and then that left you with some questions. Tell me a little bit about that.

Dr. Linda Cunningham: I was a primary care doctor, people would come to me first when they had symptoms, and oftentimes it was chest pain. A typical workup of chest pain might be an EKG, a stress test, chest x-ray, those sorts of things. If you don't find anything, and the history sounds typical, the next step is the referral to the cardiologist. A lot of those referrals then would come back after an angiogram or more sophisticated testing, like an adenosine stress test, they would come back with no ischemia. The person would come back to me and say, what now? If the person had an angiogram, I don't remember ever seeing the words myocardial bridge on the angiogram. I'm concerned now that some of those people may have had myocardial bridges that either weren't mentioned on the angiogram report or that were mentioned but were discounted as being the cause of the symptoms. Then of course, you'd send someone on to a gastroenterologist or someone else to try to figure out if it was maybe esophageal spasm or something else causing their pain. I'm just dismayed now that I may have missed people who had myocardial bridges just because of my ignorance. I looked through some of my old textbooks. There's not one mention of myocardial bridges in my internal medicine textbook or any other books that I looked through. It wasn't recognized.

JH: I know when I was on the floor of our local hospital, the cardiology floor, after an incident, I did have a heart attack. Somebody mentioned, he's got a myocardial bridge. Half the people on the floor had no clue. This is a cardiology floor. They're like, this is interesting. I was this character who was in great shape and they can't figure out why I'm having these spasms. Still, they did not correlate or wouldn't associate the bridge to the vasospasms either. That was a year ago. We're still in that space. I recall Stanford's Dr. Schnittger saying we're probably at about 35, 40% pushing 50% now, in awareness by cardiologists that these bridges do create symptoms and they need to be addressed. It was my thought, I wonder how many people actually die? Cardiac arrest looks like an occlusion from the coronary artery, but it's because of a bridge, right? We just don't know it. Which means we need to do a lot of work to get people to understand it because we can probably correct a lot of situations that need some attention. Linda, where are you currently in your process?

Dr. Linda Cunningham: I've had those preliminary tests here in town and I'm waiting for my referral to Stanford. I'm told I'm in the queue, but it may be July or August or even September before my initial visit to get the full evaluation, which I assume will be another coronary angiogram with intravenous ultrasound and the FFR testing and all of that with Dr. Tremmel.

JH: Yes, it is all that and regardless of what you've done, wherever you've done it, I think they go through the process themselves just to make sure that it's done their way. Everything I did was twice as long at Stanford than what I got prior. I thought I've already done that. I don't have to do that again. No, no. We need to do that again. And we're going to do an MRI again. We have to do that. Most of us don't like sitting in that tube and it's always an experience.

Dr. Linda Cunningham: At this point, nothing will bother me. Not even cardiac surgery will bother me because I am at the point of saying, this is not me anymore. I can't do what I want to do.

JH: I think that's really important for people to hear that it's a decision you have to make, but the alternative could be a very dire consequence. Right? We don't get to know that. You've got a great sense of humor in the situation that a lot of people really get bummed out about it and it's depressing. How do you think that's playing into your day-to-day frustration and allowing you to get through the pain when it occurs?

Dr. Linda Cunningham: I never let a moment pass without being grateful for it. We were walking this morning and we stopped and watched three downy woodpeckers on a tree because the joys of nature are so much more apparent to me now that I'm slowed down and I am able to enjoy all of that. I try to take each day, each moment at a time, be grateful for all the times I don't have chest pain. Be grateful for the fact that I can get up and walk a little bit. I've read and heard on your podcast about people who basically are bed-bound or house-bound and at least I'm not that. I can still get out a little bit and do some activity. I just try to maintain that standpoint of gratefulness for what I can do still, and gratefulness for each day, and grateful that I'm at a place where I can go to Stanford. I can go pretty much anytime I need to go. I'm grateful for being at a time when this can be dealt with. If this was 20 years ago, I probably would've said take nitro, or let's put a stent in it, or something that would've been neither helpful or very harmful. I'm happy that we're in 2023 and I'm getting diagnosed now.

JH: That's just an incredible attitude and I love it. If there was one thing from your experience to date that you would say has been most critical so far on your journey, what would you say it is?

Dr. Linda Cunningham: Making sure that I did the background work. I checked out what needed to be checked out to get myself farther along. I'm afraid if I had stuck with the advice I was getting, I would've stalled. I'm happy that I pushed things and said, no, I need more information. My husband was doing all kinds of research on the internet trying to help me out and we, together, decided that Stanford was going to be our best bet. I'm grateful, very grateful for my husband. He's a gastroenterologist. He's a primary care doctor too at times. I'm grateful for my children. Our daughter is an ICU nurse and I'm so happy that she said, I'll come out and take care of you when you have surgery or if you want me to be there at the time of surgery. I'll just drop everything and come running. Our sons have also been very supportive.

JH: That is great to hear. I want to share something from our first correspondence to give everybody a perspective of your perspective, it goes: "I'm a doctor athlete, chest pain denier, anxiety prone, myocardial bridge patient who's gone from walking seven miles a day on average in 2022 to a recliner. I've gone from fear and dreading surgery to bring it on. I've gone from believing my cardiologists to getting angry and frustrated by sheer ignorance and to trying to convince them to take it seriously. Telling them I needed more testing, telling them the best medical centers for dealing with us, trying to convince them that this should be a subject for continuing medical information at cardiology meetings."

I can't applaud that enough, Linda. I think it says everything. You're accepting it, you want to get it dealt with, and I think we all agree. We need to get the cardiology community aware that this condition is real. It creates symptoms. It can be debilitating, and at least in my opinion, I believe it can kill people.

Dr. Linda Cunningham: I actually followed up on that idea of cardiologists not getting enough education on this and I emailed the organizers of the last American College of Cardiology meetings and asked, has this subject been covered? They did have a panel discussion in March and Dr. Jennifer Tremmel was on the panel and they had a debate about whether myocardial bridges caused symptoms and what was to be done. So it is out there. People who attended the panel discussion are learning about this more.

One of the other things that has really been important to me was being taken seriously and taking myself seriously before I realized that all these chest pains were due to a bridge. I thought I was suffering from bad anxiety disorder or somaticizing, which is what we say in medicine. Some people even say it's akin to hypochondria. It's really just noticing symptoms and kind of pushing those to the forefront. Now I realize yes, I'm a little anxious, but mostly it's this, the myocardial bridge, the chest pain and the shortness of breath that were making me anxious. I would get anxious in situations where I had to speak in front of a crowd or something like that. I think a lot of it was because I would get pain. I would get pain with any sort of stressful situation, strong emotions, and oh wow, that was very, very uncomfortable. I'm trying to stay very mellow now, taking it seriously and knowing that there's a true physical problem that's causing this rather than me just being anxious. It really helps.

JH: I can't wait to follow you through the journey. I hope that you can get into Stanford sooner than later. Keep pushing.

Dr. Linda Cunningham: Yes. I'm on a first-name basis with Joy the intake coordinator. She picks up the phone and says hello, Lynn.

I'm also more than happy to be in their studies, whatever the study involves, because anything that could advance medical science is fine with me.

JH: It's frustrating to think that a cardiologist who sees it every bit as often can't accept it or see that this is really a condition that causes problems. They don't get better over time. No. They only deteriorate. I'm thrilled to have a doctor like you weigh in because you look at it from a different perspective, and if you see it from the perspective of the patient and can share it with your constituents and the other doctors, maybe that will get a little bit more attention.

Dr. Linda Cunningham: That was part of my hope. I recently discussed this with my own primary care doctor who also had not heard of myocardial bridges but educated himself about this. I said, please put the word out to everybody that this is a true cause of chest pain, exertional chest pain. It needs to be taken seriously and it needs to be evaluated with more testing than what they can do here in town. This is a condition meant for tertiary medical centers.

I was so thrilled when you said you had taken this long bike ride and you were asymptomatic and I thought of that. I hope that is me. I hope I can hike again. Hope I can go snowshoeing.

JH: With that attitude you absolutely will.

Since the interview with Linda, she has had her surgery completed at Stanford, is now living the quality of life she was accustomed to and doing what she can to continue to raise awareness of the condition while supporting others on their respective journeys.

JEREMY HESTER:
Nursing Myself To Death

(A nurse's difficult surgical decision.)

In a cruel twist of fate, our next guest found himself experiencing debilitating chest pain while on a family vacation in Hawaii, a place he had hoped would bring solace and recovery, but that wasn't to be the case.

Returning to the mainland, the pain persisted, confounding his medical colleagues and leaving him in a state of disarray. The nurse turned patient, now found himself battling a relentless adversary: uncertainty. He grappled with a debilitating condition that was shrouded in ambiguity and whose presence disrupted his professional life and family's peace of mind. His medical journey became a rollercoaster of medications, with adjustments and changes at every turn.

Jeff Holden (Host): Have we got a story for you. We've had academic doctors, PhDs. We've had doctors of medicine, MDs, and now purely coincidentally, we've got a nurse, a rather burly nurse who lives in the upper Northern California area of Redding. He's six two, around 250 pounds, 45 years old, a husband, a father of four. He suffered his first heart attack less than a year ago. It's not an anniversary most of us wish to celebrate, but it's one most of us never forget as so many of us pre-surgery have done. His mission of self-advocacy and the efforts he is going through to determine what's best for his situation is not only impressive, it may give some of you comfort knowing you're doing exactly the same thing, asking the same questions, and in many cases getting different answers. That's not all bad. We're all different people and our cases present differently, but I think we would all agree there are some standards and we have some expectations of our doctors, our cardiologists, and our surgeons.

We're going to hear the desperate attempts to minimize the pain or angina created by his myocardial bridge. This is the process to get an accurate diagnosis from where he is as he contemplates options for sternotomy or the possibility of robotic unroofing. I'm very pleased he's willing to share his progress to date as he's getting closer to a decision to finally have his unroofing surgery done.

Jeff Holden (Host): Jeremy, would you share with us what caused you to get started down this crazy, unsettling route? What happened that you knew something was wrong? You're a nurse.

Jeremy Hester (Guest): I am a nurse. I work in Northern California, as you said, in Redding. I am an ER nurse. One afternoon, going through Covid, as we all know, healthcare has been in shambles. The ER is the first place that all those shambles were happening. It's another busy day in the ER in our little, busy community and I went to have lunch and I started having a little bit of chest pressure. That was somewhere between noon and two. It was funny because I met my wife for lunch. She's also a nurse, and I met her and she saw me and she said, "You look like things aren't going well. What's going on?" "You're giving me chest pain." I joke like that, and I was having chest pain, but it wasn't your typical chest pain. It felt like the signs that we look for, crushing chest pain, shortness of breath, and I'm working super hard, so I'm already short of breath. I just kind of push it to the side, ignore it. As I was going home, walking up the driveway, my wife met me outside and she, of course, made the notation that you don't look so good. I have chest pain. She joked, "Why is it every time that you see me, you have chest pain?" Throughout that evening, we sat on the couch and I got paler, I got diaphoretic (heavily sweating), and those are not my normal ways of presenting in the evening.

She spent the next two hours trying to convince me to go to the ER. I had just left the ER. I was not going to be going back until the next morning when my shift started, and like most intelligent women, she just nodded her head or shook her head from side to side and was like, you're so dumb, but respected my decision.

About three in the morning it woke me up. The chest pain, the discomfort woke me up. The next day I go into work and I promised my wife that I would do a 12-lead EKG (a cardiac test in which 12 "leads" are attached to the body). When I got to work, one of our float nurses came by and she said, "Do you need any help with any of your patients?" I said, no. Then I suddenly remembered promising my wife, I said, actually, I need you to do a 12-lead. She said, which patient? I said, me. We went to another room. She did a quick 12-lead and my 12-lead, like most of us, it was indeterminate it, it didn't look right, but it didn't show that I was having a heart attack. It was enough, though, that my charge nurse ended up saying, you need to check in. How about we just do blood work and I'll keep working and wait for the results to come back and say that I'm dealing with a random anxiety attack and there's nothing to it? I'm making this stuff up. It's all in my head. That's where I wanted to go with it. She of course, like a good nurse leader, said, no, we're not doing that. You go and clock out. You're now a patient. So I did. We took blood work and time started flying by. The emotions, obviously because I'm healthy, were high as this is not supposed to be happening. Ultimately, in the back of my head I thought it's going to be nothing. This is all in my head. When she came back with a positive troponin, I knew I had an issue. My troponin ended up being 1.86 I believe, and that is clearly showing that something's wrong. That shocked me. I immediately started tearing up, I was like, whoa, wow, that's, that's a tough one. That was hard to face as someone who has never been really sick. We had just so happened to have our interventional cardiologist that came on that day. Someone I respect incredibly. She took me straight to the cath lab and did a cath. My cath came back completely clear. I'm going through the process in my head, like, wait, how? How is this clear? How do you connect a troponin (a cardiac muscle protein) like that to a healthy person, to having a heart attack? I don't understand. She's a very experienced interventional cardiologist and she's a fantastic doctor. She said, you have a little bit of a bridge. It's such a small bridge. I wouldn't think it would do anything. So, we're brainstorming. I'm still on the table and we're brainstorming, could I be having spasms? She said I didn't while I was in there, it didn't show that you were having any of those. The theory that we're going to go off of right now is that you have spasms. We're going to call it Prinzmetal's angina and spasms. That causes heart pain.

JH: Kudos to her because that's something that so many docs miss. They just dismiss it before they even have the discussion. Not only did she point out to you that you've got a bridge and the identification it's a relatively short bridge, she went right into the spasm discussion, that's a perfect progression. It's great to hear.

Jeremy Hester: To be honest, it's pretty amazing. She explained to me that she's had a few patients like this in the past, and ultimately most of 'em resolve on their own. She told me to expect within two to three months that things will get better. She's had about five patients in her career who stumped her. Which is a pretty good number considering those are low stats, which is great for her, but I was one of them, and so immediately she gave me, I believe it was amlodipine and she gave me aspirin and sublingual nitroglycerin. And she said, whenever the pain starts, take a sublingual and over the next few months it'll resolve. So I knew I was going to be off for a few weeks. My family decided to take a holiday. I grew up in Hawaii. We decided to go back and just try to relax as much as possible. We immediately left and went to Hawaii and visited my family there.

The problem was it wasn't relaxing. My chest pain got worse and the day we were leaving, my ankles, all of a sudden my lower legs just blew up. They swelled up and the chest pain got worse and new, symptoms were happening to the point where it was scary.

JH: To be clear, you had not had surgery yet? You still have angina. You still have the chest pains. They've progressed. They've gotten a little bit worse as they tend to do once these symptoms present, because the compression of the artery from the bridge doesn't improve until something causes it to improve.

Jeremy Hester: Right. To bring that story to a close, we came home. In that period of time, it was about 10 days, I went through a bottle and a half of Nitro in 10 days. Taking the Nitro, besides the wonderful headache, it will relieve the chest pain briefly, and I didn't understand. What I did know was that angina or the spasms were related potentially to stress. So fast forward, I come back to the states and fly into Sacramento. We talked to the interventional cardiologist and she informed me that is not normal. That I should probably go ahead and go to the hospital and she'd already talked to the doctors there at UC Davis, which is a great facility. But my concern was if I go into the ER and I don't have elevated troponin, they're just going to kick me to the street. They're going to say my labs are normal. Go home. I went back to our home in Redding, having chest pain the whole way trying to find some kind of place of peace to try to somehow will the pain back into a place of not having pain.

I go back to the ER, have my labs drawn, and they were fine. I had a new symptom: when I would lean forward, it would hurt. When I'd lean back, it was fine. From my education I knew that could potentially be pericarditis. I asked for tests for that. At the end of the day, I got discharged. You're fine. Nothing's wrong, let's change your medicine. Let's get you off of amlodipine. That's actually when we started the whole process of knowing that it wasn't going to get better over the next two to three months. It surprised the interventional cardiologist. She said, this is outside of my wheelhouse. Let's get you to a specialist. She put two requests in, one to Davis and one to Stanford. My insurance didn't cover Davis, but it did cover Stanford. Problem was, I couldn't work. I could hardly get up. The pain would just start almost immediately in the day. Sometimes it would wake me up first thing, and there was no real rhyme or reason. Sometimes it would hurt in the afternoon. Sometimes it would hurt in the morning. It wasn't super clear. We switched medicine. I changed to sublingual nitroglycerin. Instead of taking it all the time, I changed to just taking it when I needed it. We changed from the amlodipine to a low-dose Cardizem. It seemed to help a little bit, but in all of these medicines, everything seemed to help a little bit, but not enough. Not even enough to where I could bear it. This is still terrible. And then you had the side effects of the medicine.

The Cardizem seemed to work a little bit. Then what did we do? Aspirin. Amlodipine, got off. Oh, and then they started me on the iso or big mono Iso sorbate mononitrate, the long acting Nitro. The doc said, you can't keep taking this sublingual like this. That was good. It took me about two weeks to adjust. When I'd get out of bed, I would almost fall down because of the dizziness because my blood pressure was so low. Each one of these medicines that were added, each time that we added a different dose to the medicine, I would have about a two week adjustment period. It's discouraging because I didn't have the answer.

JH: It was just a remedy?

Jeremy Hester: Yes. I'm a nurse in Western medicine, but I don't want to take medicines. I don't want to be reliant on these medicines my whole life. That did not sound good to me. They weren't even working. Finally, I heard back from Stanford. I heard back from them and they let me know that they would totally see me. We went straight to one of their specialists, Dr. Jennifer Tremmel. She and her team are fantastic, but the soonest they could get me in was April, which was like five or six months, seven months away. Which sounded terrible to me. I'm going to lose my job.

JH: You also don't know that you're not going to have a heart attack.

Jeremy Hester: Totally. Let's talk about a mix of emotions. I want to live, but I also want my family to eat. This is tough. I'm super thankful that they were able to get me in a couple months early, they called me out of the blue and I'm home, feeling terrible, feeling useless. For whatever it's worth, I was feeling super demasculinized. I went to one of our local cardiologists. I knew I needed a cardiologist, so I went to the cardiologist and this is where my story melds in with everyone else's. The cardiologist was completely dismissive. We sat down and he came in the door and he said, well, I've looked at your cath and it says you're clear, so don't worry about it. I said, I was told by the interventional cardiologist that it's probably spasms. I said, I had a heart attack, so explain it. He just shrugged his shoulders. He's like, I don't know, but you've got 10 years. I was like, what do you mean I've got 10 years? He said it takes 10 years for plaque to form in an artery enough to kill you. You're going to be fine for at least 10 years. Yeah. That is not an okay answer. What I said was, your answer isn't satisfactory. He said, well, to be honest, I don't know. I said, cool, I just needed this to have a cardiologist. I'll keep my appointment with Stanford. It was a shrug of the shoulders and thanks for your copay and goodbye. It is how it felt and it's been really encouraging to read so many people's stories on the support group because I'm not alone. I was pretty disappointed, obviously, and at this point really frustrated. Then, of course, he's saying I'm fine. There's nothing wrong. I'm thinking it might be in my head, but there's this thing of me having a heart attack. That is keeping me in the game. I'm still having pain every day, literally every day.

JH: It's debilitating to the point where you can't go to work?

Jeremy Hester: Yes. It was awful.

JH: There are so many people who I can envision nodding their heads from your first opening discussion of the drug therapy, the type of drugs you're getting. They're going yep, got that. Yep. Chest pain. Nope. Won't go away. Now it's debilitating. Nope. Can't work. To the point, oh, now I'm being dismissed by a cardiologist. Been there, done that. Finally, I've got somebody who at least understands and acknowledges that I do have something and I have an appointment to see them. I can't wait.

Jeremy Hester: Yes. It was the interventional cardiologist who did my initial cath. I feel like it was almost a godsend, or it was a godsend for me personally, the fact that she had my back on it was amazing.

JH: She saved you a whole lot of time.

Jeremy Hester: Wow. My journey has been so discouraging in so many ways, yet it is so minimal compared to what everyone else on this group has been going through. I count my blessings in that.

Jeff Holden: Now you're off to Stanford.

Jeremy Hester: Yes.

Jeff Holden: For your provocative test with Dr. Tremmel?

Jeremy Hester: Yes. I travel to Stanford and it's a different level and I'm in healthcare. I've worked at hospitals and Stanford is next level for sure. The professionalism of everyone from the bottom up. It was an amazing experience.

I sit down with Dr. Tremmel's physician assistant, we spent some time, and then Dr. Tremmel came in and the appointment was amazing. She confirmed, she said, how did you feel like a kid? Were you short of breath? I was very active. I was a big soccer player, a big football player, and I was in shape as a young kid. She said, I bet you thought it was normal. I said, yeah. It's not normal. Now I'm starting to connect the dots. Wow. In a 10 minute conversation, she pinpointed all of the things that I dismissed as a young person, young adult, up until now, as being a normal thing. She said, it sounds like you qualify for more extensive testing, so if you're up for it, let's do it. So we did. I came back and I did the cath with the extensive testing and the acetylcholine and the dobutamine and I looked up at one point, I saw my heart rate was 144. Dr. Tremmel, I could hear her and she asked, Mr. Hester, are you doing okay? I said, I don't know what you just gave me, but if you don't stop, you're gonna kill me.

JH: Was that not the most unusual experience to be lying still? You feel your heart go from a resting heart rate to more, to more, to more, to more, to the most exertion you could ever put on it? I told her as a cyclist, I feel like I'm climbing the steepest hill I've ever climbed and I'm lying here looking at you. It's like, is this really happening?

Jeremy Hester: Yeah. I'm not running a treadmill, I'm not running a hill. Right. I remember saying it and she said, okay. But it felt like my teeth were going to explode. Anyway, that procedure was done and I had to recover for several hours and make sure I was good.

JH: What they're doing for the people who have not had this provocative testing is they're diagnosing not only the severity of the spasm because they have flow meters in your artery at that point, but they're also diagnosing the flow forward and backward under stress and rest. And not to get technical in terms of what they call it, but that's the detail of what they're trying to get out of that test. Right?

Jeremy Hester: Yes. At the end of the day, they came out and I was hoping for one or the other. Unfortunately, I was told that I had, the words that were used very specifically, I have severe diffuse coronary artery spasms, and I have a significant bridge. That was disappointing.

JH: But also, and I'm not going to put words in your mouth, was it not comforting to know, all right, now at least we know, we know what's causing this? The uncertainty of it is over. We know this is what these symptoms are, they're being caused by this bridge. And at least I'm one step closer to some resolution.

Jeremy Hester: Yes. Yes. If you take away my propensity to want to live in this reality that nothing's wrong,

JH: It's called denial, which we all do.

Jeremy Hester: Totally. Absolutely.

JH: For some reason, I don't know why it's so difficult for us to say I had a heart attack.

Jeremy Hester: Yeah. I don't like that at all.

JH: I still struggle saying I had a heart attack. How did I have a heart attack? I took care of myself. Right? I heard you say it, and I'm sure a lot of other people are there and we laugh about it. It's a reality. We have to accept the fact that it happened. The reality is it's not our image of a person who has a heart attack. Typically, no matter who you are, no matter what you look like, if you had that heart attack, the person you look at in the mirror isn't the person who was supposed to have a heart attack.

Jeremy Hester: That's right.

JH: But we have to address it. Fortunately, the good news is we do get to live with the history of the fact that we had that heart attack. Because there are other people who have it and don't.

Jeremy Hester: They decided to put me on, what was it? I think Bystolic. The beta blocker. I can't remember exactly, but-wait, they changed the medicine. That's what it was. They changed it to something else and I responded well. There's hope at the time we might be able to manage this without doing surgery. Of course you want to go with a less aggressive route. They came to me and part of me was like, no, let's just cut it out. Let's just go to surgery. It'll fix everything and I'll get back to a normal life. I don't have to be on these stupid meds my whole life. That's how I feel about it. I don't want to. What happens if the medication factory burns down and I can't find the meds, I'm going to die. That sucks. All these thoughts and all these fears and my mind just starts dancing and I can't sleep because I'm thinking about it. Well, I guess we should try it with the meds. Like all the other medications, they worked for a time and then they stopped working. It wasn't giving me the quality of life, and so we spent the next few months, every two weeks I would have a phone appointment with Stanford, with Shannon, Dr. Tremmel's, PA. It was fantastic, amazing care. We would talk about it, we'd talk about my symptoms, then we would talk about the potential medicines that we could change. We quite literally were practicing medicine by adjusting the pharmaceuticals. How long do I wait before it's actually causing damage? These are the thoughts that are going on and to the point where we even tried antipsychotics, anti-depressants.

JH: I appreciate you saying that because a lot of people don't even want to address that. There may be somebody who has symptoms. That might help them. Absolutely. We don't know what's the root cause of this. Not everybody's symptoms are caused by the same thing. Right? To the point of many cardiologists, a lot of bridges are benign, they could be triggered by something. I appreciate the fact that you did bring that up.

I'm going to push you along to the next step there. You went that route and you said, maybe there's an organic route I can go.

Jeremy Hester: I was so frustrated. A doctor friend of mine sent me a few articles from the NIH that were CBDs effects on endothelial inflammation in rats. I want to not die, really. It's not something I, per se, believe in on a personal level, but I was so frustrated. I was willing to do anything, so

I went and got some gummies and trial and error, and lo and behold, it worked every time. I didn't have any pain. I would take the gummy and in about 30 minutes pain was gone—and this is in combination with the other medications I was on. It was very encouraging on one hand for me, they could control the pain. It was the first time I had a string of painless days since the whole thing started in August and it worked for four days. On the fourth day, it stopped working and went back to what it was before, just like all the other medicine. Talking with Shannon, she says, "Well, Jeremy, we were at the limit of exhausting the medicine. It might be time to start talking about surgery." All of a sudden, the reality of that scared me.

Wait a minute. I know I wanted it before but getting my chest opened up is really scary for me. I asked if we could try adding a beta blocker to the calcium channel blocker. Generally, they don't want to do that because the effects on the heart rate and your blood pressure are really bad. So we added a low dose of that. The combination of what I've been doing has given me the best results so far, but I still can't walk a block. I still can't exercise. When I'm sitting here on the couch talking to you, it doesn't hurt for the first time in eight months, which is a positive. But it's not a way to live.

JH: It's exertional under this particular medical regime?

Jeremy Hester: It's both. If there's an increasing anxiety, it'll cause it to happen.

JH: I'm glad that your anxiety must be fairly low doing this conversation because you haven't had an episode in the duration of it so far, so that's great.

Jeremy Hester: Yeah, I actually have, I've had a little bit of chest pain, but I've gotten to where I ignore it. I try to ignore it. We fast forward and, and we start talking about needing surgery.

We set up an appointment. As so many people are aware, Stanford has the leading research for myocardial bridges and in Dr. Boyd, one of the leading surgeons. So we had an appointment with Dr. Jack Boyd, but I was like, do I qualify? I'm not sure if I qualify. I don't know. Are we having this meeting to determine whether I qualify? So my understanding going down there was like, oh no, you do qualify. Ultimately, I'm not as bad as some, but I have a decrease in distal perfusion from my bridge. I definitely qualified for the surgery. And then the severe spasms, that's a whole different story. Which I guess is pretty bad too from the pictures I saw.

JH: Endothelial dysfunction is no fun.

Jeremy Hester: No, and it's hard because I try to narrow it down. When is my bridge being activated and when are my spasms being activated? I have different pains, sometimes it's dull and it goes on for a while. Sometimes I feel like someone just took a little needle right into my heart. So I had the meeting with Dr. Boyd and his PA, which was again, fantastic. He really took the time to explain things, go over the pictures, to talk about the potential fears of surgery, and to give me time to really think about it. And you know, I had questions where I'm like, I'm wanting to nail you down on some of these questions. He's a great surgeon. He shares I can't nail him down on those because there are a lot of unknowns still. Right? One of the things that is said is, what is a correlation between endothelial dysfunction, the spasms? What is a correlation between the spasms and the bridge? If you unroof me successfully and you fix the bridge, is that going to fix the spasms? The short answer I got was that there's not a guarantee. There seems to be a correlation, but there are no studies that have been done to connect the two. We think there's a correlation, but again, we can't put our name to the fact that there are or there aren't, and that's honest.

JH: For those of us on the other side of this conversation right now, hearing you speak, where you are, not unroofed yet, you're pre-surgery. Yes, we're going, yes. There's a connection. It does work. It does minimize the spasms. Totally.

Jeremy Hester: I know, but what if I'm that one guy? Right? Even asking Dr. Boyd, how many people die on the table? None. And what if I'm the first, right?

You know what I mean? Those fears. I've had a couple surgeries. Do I respond well? I don't respond great. Do I respond terribly? No, I'm still here. I play that kind of devil's advocate sometimes where I think, what if?

The consult went like everything I've had at Stanford, amazing. They were incredibly professional. They took the time. I didn't feel like they were rushing. These are busy people. These are world-renowned specialists and they've got other people to see, and I didn't feel like I was rushed or dismissed. It felt good. It felt really good. He was honest. This could help. Maybe it won't. But it could. The percentages are pretty good with patients who've had it saying that it does help. And so that started the process of, okay, okay, we have to do the surgery. He's actually the one who told me to come on the support group. He said, I hear there's a support group. It might be really helpful. It's a four-and-a-half-hour drive from Stanford to my home without traffic. I went on, joined the group and I spent probably two hours for the drive, reading stories, reading test results, reading, testimonies, crying on several occasions because, holy moly, their story is like mine. I've been dismissed by a cardiologist and a good one at that, and told, we don't know, something's going on. It might be spasms. Here I am wondering am I making this up? Is this in my head? It's not in my head, but is this in my head? We don't know what it is. I met with Dr. Boyd and the big question now was, okay, when? When are we doing the surgery? Dr. Boyd was pretty straightforward. At that point, the option was sternotomy. I'm a little nervous and I shouldn't be because I'm going to take care of it, and then it's Stanford, it's Dr. Boyd, I'm going to be fine. There was still fear there. Reading as much as I could, all of a sudden I start reading, do robotics, try robotics. If robotics is an option in your area, do robotics. Stanford doesn't do robotics yet. This surgery alone is new. It's a new heart surgery that hasn't been around very long and robotics is even newer than that. I don't know what the data is, but it's so new. There isn't enough information on whether it's the way to go or not.

That's scary. It was enough to play on my fears, enough to play on my concerns. Medically, from the surgical site, recovery is stated to be about three months. Somewhere between three and six months is what I'm told. Everyone I started hearing from in the group, and I understand you have to filter things in the group because there are a lot of things that are said that you know, that's not a thing.

JH: Everybody is different. There are no two of us alike in any way, shape, or form and our deformities are different. The process to fix us is different, and again, no two are alike. Even our chemical makeup is different. Right? How we present is different. The way our hormones produce is different, so it's very hard and frustrating for somebody to put out a blanket statement. No, it's not really like that. To the point of, I hear you very, very clearly stating, you know your body pretty well. You understand it well. For those who do, they're going to come out much better on the other side of this thing than those who don't and just try to motor through and get resolved and maybe don't understand all the nuances of the entire process, right?

I want to get you from the sternotomy discussion because we spent a fair amount of time on that, to the robotics. I understand everybody's concern when they think, okay, this is faster, I'll be back to work. I don't have to worry about lifting as much because that's my job, right? There's also that fear of this sternotomy and I'm being cut open versus this robotic thing that I don't get opened up as much. You've done some extremely powerful self-advocacy on this because not only have you vetted Dr. Boyd's process and Stanford's process, but you've now actually had a conversation with another doctor who does robotic surgery, correct?

Jeremy Hester: Yes. I spoke with both his team and him. I started doing research and there were several, really only a handful, but for me, a list of three to four surgeons who did robotics. They did id the unroofing robotic approach that I potentially was interested in based on primarily, honestly, based on people in the group. I started looking into their numbers, their websites, their reputations, and I settled on Dr. Husam Balkhy at the University of Chicago. Knowing that he's one of the leaders in robotics, knowing that his numbers for this procedure were significantly lower than Dr. Boyd's, I still dug deeper.

JH: Dr. Boyd is pushing more than 12 years of doing these.

Jeremy Hester: Yes. Right. I did speak both to the nurse practitioner of Dr. Balkhy yesterday, it was a consult that was very similar to Dr. Boyd's, very professional. They answered my questions thoroughly and we were able to have a Zoom call. They're in Chicago, I'm in California. It was a great conversation. A lot of questions were answered. And mind you, because I'm in healthcare, I have access to surgeons. It's a tough one because the robotics and the traditional approaches aren't enemies, but they're not friends. Some of the old-school docs would say no. Robotics is not experienced enough. That's true. It's not got the history of success the sternotomy does. The fear for me was …Mmm. Do I go with the sure hand and potentially lose my job because the recovery is going to be so long that I don't have job security?

That was my big fear. I've already taken enough time off of work and now I've had to go back to work to keep from losing my job and to keep my insurance and, that process that I'm sure everyone is having to go through to one degree or another. I'm back at work having to pop nitro all the time to ride this real fine line of having another heart attack. I need to work so that I can have insurance to have a surgery to potentially save my life. It's a tough, tough road, right? It's not as bad as some, but we all have different paths to walk. One of the biggest allures of doing robotics is recovery time.

I'm wanting to share my process as I'm going through this because I haven't made the decision yet on which one. I have the sure hand the amazing experience at Stanford. They're an absolutely professional group of people who are definitely the leaders in myocardial bridges and know what to do and know how to fix it. I have no doubt, but my big fear is the recovery time. With my job that's going to be a bit to be able to do what I do.

With the robotics, one of the questions that I had that a surgeon posted to me was they don't have the angle, the angle going through the chest. They do five punctures through the ribs and one's a chest tube and the other one is the camera, right? With my chest cavity, how do you get over the heart? When you do a sternotomy that is right over the heart, that's hands in and the approach is good. I'm having to weigh that angle, does it give a good view? I'm hearing one thing on one side, I'm hearing another thing on the other side. How much of that is just preference? That's how I look at it in the world as such a new way of doing it.

Now, the numbers that I gathered are good on both and the risks, there are pros and cons for both. One of the big questions I had is, give me your percentages, give me your numbers. The problem is they don't have enough. We're not really comparing apples to apples. Whether that's Dr. Boyd or Dr. Balkhy or any of the other doctors who do robotics, they have done other heart surgeries with robotics. I don't want to be your first. No, thank you. I don't want to be your second either, you know what I mean? I have options and I know that probably comes across as a kick in the pants for some people, because a lot of them would just love to have a surgeon that would say, yes.

JH: Agreed.

Jeremy Hester: I don't want to take away from anybody who's walking through that because my heart goes out to you. That's awful. I've been blessed, I have a choice. I'm taking that very seriously. Very thankfully, it's not lost on me. I have a choice. It doesn't take away the fear, it doesn't take away that this is still heart surgery. I'm still in the middle of making the choice, but the choice right now is a more experienced team in dealing with unroofing that is close by, or do I travel across the country and have the less invasive, quicker recovery surgery? The one thing I can definitely say that I'm gathering from the different people I've reached out to is no matter what, have the surgery.

JH: Yes.

Jeremy Hester: The thing that the people who are struggling with, like me, the people that are really struggling back and forth with making the choice of do you have robotics? Do you have a sternotomy or a thoracotomy, whichever route that you're choosing, we can assuredly say, I can gather this, and I feel like pretty confidently from the people that have had it, do it no matter the approach because it's going to improve your life. That's not medical, that's just what seems to be what everyone says.

JH: There is a consensus that the surgery does improve the quality of life. Post-surgery. Period. End of story. It doesn't always minimize all the symptoms or eradicate the symptoms, but it certainly gives you the ability to get the majority of the life you knew previously, back. Right? Even if you have to take some small dosage of medication, it's far better than it was previously.

Jeremy Hester: If I have the procedure in Chicago, I'm not going to my local hospital.

JH: To your point, everybody doesn't have the luxury of that option. It may be their local hospital's willing to give it a shot and try it. Which may still be better than the consequence of living without it because at some point the bridge will further restrict the vessel. It happens over time. As we age, it continues to weaken, weaken, weaken, and at some point it can't reflex back and the flow is diminished to the point of severity. Maybe a heart attack again, another heart attack, or a severe heart attack. I think any option of a choice to do or not to do is far better than no choice or no option. And because so many do have the, we'll call it the luxury of choice to robotic versus sternotomy, it's a great discussion and it's great for people to hear somebody who's going through that in their mind right now. You've explained extremely well, both sides, you know the things to be aware of, the things that are going through your mind, the challenges, mentally, that you have to go through the machinations of, oh, well, this, this, this, this. Then, the other side of your brain goes, well, what about this, this, this, this? And. You have that extra burden of weight of your work, your job.

Jeremy Hester: Well, that's the risk we're taking and that that is honestly where the minimally invasive approach has an allure. I started down that path, quelling my fears, and so it's one of those things where if you want the sure thing and if you want a sure hand, I will recommend Stanford, even though it hasn't happened yet, but based on my experience with their numbers. That said, you have many people out there saying, yeah, we got this. Did you do the testing? The best testers on this right now are Stanford. Right? They know their thing. It comes back to a level of faith. At the end of the day, my health isn't in my hands. I'm going to have to trust a higher power. I do. You've got to put your faith in something.

Jeremy, ultimately did choose Dr. Balkhy at University of Chicago to perform robotic surgery. After a bout or two with pericarditis, I'm pleased to say his symptoms have been greatly diminished, he was back to work within weeks and he continues to do well and has returned to doing most of what he did prior to his surgery. His trust in a higher power and his faith led him down the right path for his situation.

SARAH MILLER & VERONICA THAXTON: When Too Much Becomes Too Much

(Two very athletic women, a distance runner and a triathlete, share their stories.)

Six and a half weeks after her heart surgery, Veronica Thaxton, a triathlete, found herself on a journey from triathlon training to confronting the reality of unexpected heart distress symptoms. Her determination to uncover the truth about her health led her to discover a myocardial bridge, a journey that details the frustration of being initially dismissed and the power of persistence.

Alongside Veronica, Sarah Miller, a marathon runner, paints a vivid picture of emotional resilience amid misdiagnoses, culminating in her heart surgery that brought clarity and relief after years of uncertainty. Veronica, and Sarah's stories reveal the relentless pursuit of accurate diagnosis and the life-changing impact of finding healthcare professionals who truly listen and act. Their experiences serve as a testament to the importance of seeking multiple opinions, trusting one's instincts, and understanding the power of community support in overcoming medical challenges.

Jeff Holden (Host): Veronica, you're now not even seven weeks out from surgery, and Sarah, you're about a year-and-a-half out from surgery, could you each walk us through what occurred that got you to the point that you realized something was wrong?

Veronica Thaxton (Guest): I've been an athlete for most of my life and a triathlete since 2000. Beginning of 2021, I was training for an "ultra", for a race, just a run. I started the year with some pretty heavy training, went straight from that and training for a half-Ironman and completed that in June and then straight into training for half-Ironman World Championships in September. Beginning in August 2021, I started having some left-side chest pain but nothing too significant, yet I certainly noticed it: sharp shooting pain that would come and go. It lasted for a couple of weeks and I thought I was about due for a checkup with my internist and get some blood work done. I'm really careful when I'm training, especially at a high level anyway, to have that monitored and tracked. I saw my internist about three weeks into August and told him of this chest pain I was having and the day it started. In addition to the chest pain, that really wasn't too worrisome at the time, I started having some pressure on the left side of my chest. Hadn't experienced it before. Still hard to describe, it was more than just someone pushing in on your chest, just a very strange sensation. My training didn't feel as good and of course, as an athlete you think, why am I so tired? Am I sleeping? Am I over-training? All these questions athletes ask when the performance isn't where it should be. I couldn't figure anything out. That day that I got the chest pressure I thought, oh man, something is not right.

The visit to my internist didn't really go very well and I know a lot of people share the same story. He told me what many others have heard: it's all in your head, it's some anxiety. He was a triathlete and had known me for years. He ordered a chest X-ray, and he did the EKG and calcium-scoring CT. All of that was fine. "You're fit as a fiddle. Your stress is probably too high. I know your job is busy. It must be in your head; stress and anxiety." I just couldn't accept that. I've got a busy job. I didn't feel like it was taking a toll on me, mentally, though, or physically, and didn't really know what to do next, but left there thinking all right, maybe I need some sleep and this feeling will go away. From the end of October till September, I was just able to do less and less, until I could barely go for a walk. I came from training at a high level for a half ironman to barely being able to walk, came home one day from a walk with just the classic heart attack symptoms, chest pain, radiating at my neck and down my arm, and unable to walk and hard to breathe. I called my friend who's a nurse, and she said go to the ER. So I went, and you know you get the same thing there, a chest X-ray and EKG and another CT. On the CT at the ER, they said that well, we think there might be something there. It's inconclusive for blockages, so we think you need a heart cath. I did that on the next day, on September 10th. Just three or four weeks from nothing to something really bad. The heart cath indicated I had a myocardial bridge. Okay, so what do I do? They said nothing. They said these are common, they're benign, and sent me home the next day with just a prescription for my calcium channel blocker and a statin which I didn't need. When I asked, well, when can I run? "Oh well, you know, give it a week, you'll be fine." They just clearly didn't know what to do with me. I'm young and fit and healthy. The whole two days I was there, there were people, doctors and nurses, peeking in the window to look at this athlete who had this heart thing going on, and they just shrugged their shoulders and said all right, thanks for stopping by, you'll be fine.

I went home and over the next couple of weeks started feeling worse. The pressure was intensifying, I was getting more left-side chest pain. So I went back to the cardiologist I had seen in the hospital, and he started treating me for pericarditis, thinking, "Well, you know, your troponins were elevated, you had some fluid around your heart, let's treat you for pericarditis." It didn't work, kept feeling worse and went back to him a few weeks later and he said, "Well, you know, it looks like it may be the bridge." He'd already told me that you don't stent the bridge. He's done it once in 30 years. It's very risky because the stents can fracture. At this point he said well, it looks like it's your bridge, maybe we should stent it. I left and got a second opinion.

JH: Get another cardiologist. You don't stent a bridge.

Veronica Thaxton: Absolutely, and there's a lot of talk about that on the Facebook page which I like. I think the first thing that we do is when they say you have a myocardial bridge, you Google it. I found Stanford's site and I read about stenting it and what to do and what not to do. I thought, no, I'm not going to listen to any more of this. I'm going to get a second opinion and the second opinion cardiologist I'm sure others will relate to this too. They get referrals to these great, highly respected, very credentialed and experienced cardiologists and they can't help you and that's what I ran into. A second time. He told me three things. Eventually, after more tests and an MRI check for pericarditis, he said, well, three things. One, you had something going on, and he was referring to pericarditis. It was an explanation for the mysterious pain. You had something going on, you're getting better and you're just afraid to work out. I said really, because I couldn't walk from the parking lot to the office and right now, just sitting here, my chest hurts and there's pressure and it's hard to breathe. He told me it was in my head. I went home discouraged and I'm embarrassed and ashamed to say that. I started to doubt myself and think well, maybe this is in my head, maybe I did have something going on and I've built this up, and maybe I really am afraid to push myself. I did what any athlete in denial of having a problem would do. On my walk the next day I started to run a little bit, a minute or two at a time, and I'd walk a little bit more, another minute or two at a time. That worked for a couple of days, but on the third day I did that, I couldn't walk. Horrible chest pain, horrible pressure, ended up back in the ER that night and when they called that cardiologist, he never returned the call. They didn't know what to do with me. I never heard back from him and I thought this is crazy.

By this point it was April, so this started in August 21. By April 22, I was still unable to do anything and just frustrated and not getting better. I thought, okay, that's two cardiologists, they don't know what to do with me. Maybe it really is just a bad case of pericarditis that won't heal. I'm going to go see a congenital heart disease guy and see if it is the bridge or not. I found one in town. He didn't really have experience with these. He'd seen them, of course, but never had a symptomatic patient and so I told him what was going on and he said well, let's do a cardiopulmonary exercise test. I did that in June of 22. And I just couldn't walk. I got worse.

JH: You're all the way to June, seven months, almost eight months later, nine months of concern, having symptoms that even appeared to be heart attack-like?

Veronica Thaxton: Yes, all the classic heart attack symptoms, the pressure and the pain and the shortness of breath and you know, down the left arm, up the neck and all of that. I was patient when they told me, oh, it's just pericarditis not healing, I tried to believe that and well, you have to give it time and medicine. I did have a follow up with him and he said I think you may need to see a rheumatologist. So I did, in November, and I talked to the rheumatologist. I never even took a seat. I think he came in talking about how I probably needed to be on some anti-rheumatic drugs, even though I didn't have symptoms. He was checking me for joint swelling and dry eyes and all of these things and still telling me that I needed to be on prednisone and hydroxychloroquine. You've got to listen to your gut instinct and I should have done that several times in this process. One time when I did was when he was telling me all these things and I said this is not right, this is not the problem, this is something wrong with my heart. I didn't go back to that internist for a while, not until I needed some routine labs done.

Sarah Miller (Guest): We want to hear what they're telling us. It's fine, we can go out and do our things, we're good, it's all in our head and so we think, okay, then I'll go push harder because I can push.

Veronica Thaxton: Yes, I'm an athlete, I can push. If I've gotten in a little funk in my head mentally, I can get out of that. Exactly.

JH: So you got through that June rheumatoid doc who's trying to say you have some sort of arthritic situation. And what then?

Veronica Thaxton: I just completely dismissed him because what he was saying was just so contradictory. He said many other things that just didn't add up. I thought, no, it's my heart, it's not a rheumatological problem. Yeah, and after that exercise stress test, I felt continuously worse for several days after. When I called my cardiologist back, they had planned to do the FFR (fractional flow reserve, a minimally invasive procedure) CT, but it was going to take a few weeks for insurance to approve that. I call back asking if this is normal after the exercise test. I can't even walk now. They said, no, it's not, go to the ER, we're going to get that CT done and we're going to figure this out. They sent me there. I showed up, they did the FFR CT and they said it's your bridge. Yeah, it took from August 21 till June of 22, to get a definitive answer. In hindsight I wish I would have done things differently and pushed more towards the bridge. But when you're being told it's so rare to have symptoms, then you go with the experts. I think what we're going to learn now is that they still say it's very rare to be symptomatic from a bridge. I think we're going to learn that it's not rare that all of these people who've taken so long to get a correct diagnosis and are being told that it's in their head or it's another problem. It's rare to get the correct diagnosis. When I got that diagnosis, my cardiologist didn't quite know what to do with me because he'd not seen anyone symptomatic before. First, he told me that surgery was not an option because it was deep. The measurements they gave me initially were 1.8 centimeters long and about four millimeters deep. He said it goes right up to the cavity of the ventricle. Surgery is not an option; it'd be too risky. I said am I going to live like this my entire life? Will I ever be able to run? He said, no, you won't be able to. And yes, this is how you're going to live. I didn't accept that. I said no and he said, well, give me a few weeks, let me figure something out. I said okay, got home from the hospital and started downloading all my labs and ordering the CDs and as soon as I got those, I sent my records off to Stanford, Chicago and Cleveland Clinic and I knew pretty much that Stanford was where I wanted to go. I'd read enough over the 10 months to know that Stanford was the place to be. With their experience and being the worldwide leaders in this, I thought that's where I need to get myself, at least get my records and have them reviewed and see what they have to say.

JH: I'll make the assumption you then had the provocative test at Stanford and they redid everything that you've already had done. They did it their way, and at that point they identified your situation and said here's what we can do.

Veronica Thaxton: Yes. There was a long waiting list. I guess they do one bridge surgery a week, so they receive my records beginning in July. Of course, it takes some time for Dr. Schnittger who does reviews on her own time. It took about six weeks to be able to look at mine. And they said sign up for testing, gave me a surgery slot. I went back at the beginning of February, first week of February, for testing, and yeah, you're right. They redid the CT and they found at Stanford that it was about twice as long as they initially told me and that it went into the cavity of the ventricle. Not just that it was deep, right up to it, but it went into the ventricle. And I had two bridges, so testing there was much different from the results.

Sarah Miller: Wow, I really want to cry. I feel like it makes me so sad that they were okay to just say you have to live like that.

Veronica Thaxton: My cardiologist did come around. When he said, give me a few weeks, I gave him a few weeks. I sent my records on anyway. Then I got a call from Mayo Clinic in Rochester. He had sent my records there and they called to offer me a surgery date in December, beginning of December 22. Boy that sounded tempting. You know how it is when you're feeling bad, you just want to be fixed. I talked to them and I listened, but I didn't feel comfortable with the testing that they were going to do, or really the lack of testing, and with what they were agreeing to. They were offering me surgery really based on what I felt like was an incomplete view of my records. They hadn't even seen everything that I had done, and it was tempting. But I thought, if this is deep, I want to go to

Stanford, I want to go where there's experience and knowledge, and I'm glad I waited. It was really hard to wait that extra time, but, gosh, it was still worth it, especially knowing that it was more significant than what I originally thought. I'm glad I waited. It was scheduled for Valentine's Day. I was really excited about getting my heart fixed on Valentine's Day. I've had my heart broken on Valentine's Day. I've never had my heart fixed on Valentine's Day. But I had had some Pectus Excavatum (a birth defect of the formation of the sternum) that needed to be corrected in addition to the unroofing. Dr. Boyd, the day before surgery, said "Let's hold off. I want to talk to the thoracic surgeon and the radiologist to get the measurements for the Pectus." So, they decided that I did need a correction. We put it off until February 16th. That was my surgery day. I had the unroofing by Dr Boyd and the modified Ravitch procedure by Dr. Berry.

Sarah Miller: Do you have any other heart conditions?

Veronica Thaxton: No, no other heart conditions.

JH: Sarah, you're actually teeing us up for a beautiful segue here, because yours is a little bit of a different story in terms of what led you to your actual surgery. So go ahead.

Sarah Miller: Mine started a long time ago, in 2013. It was kind of up and down. I was having issues, I would go to the doctor, they would do tests. Ultimately, they said it's in your head. They did a stress test, they did multiple, multiple tests and this is 2013. I went to breathing doctors and cardiologists between 2013 and 2018, stress tests and finally, the breathing tests doctor looked at me and said your next stop needs to be at the psychologist. I jokingly but not jokingly, pushed back. I said, okay, well, I'm going to prove them wrong. I'm going to push harder, I'm going to train longer, I'm going to, you know, all of the things that we do. And in 2019, I went out for a run. I knew I was not feeling well. I started up Costco Hill and it's a pretty significant hill in our area and I thought, oh, I'm just tired. I've been traveling. I feel like I'm going to faint, I feel heavy. My chest is really heavy. I started feeling like, oh, I need to maybe go to the bathroom, just all of these feelings. I said to my friend who was running with me I'm going to jump into this outhouse really quick and she said okay. The next thing I know I'm outside the outhouse on the ground, waking up, and I had completely passed out, hit my head and had to be taken to the hospital in an ambulance. There, we get to the emergency room and I have a concussion and I'm clearly having some heart pain and my whole left side is heavy. It's tingly. The doctor comes in and says, you've had a heart attack. We're keeping you and walks out of the room and my husband and I are sitting there, and we look at each other and I'm like, there's no way. There's no way I've had a heart attack. They kept me there for a couple of days. They did multiple tests. My troponin levels just kept rising, rising, rising. They would not let me leave until they started going down. Finally, they did. That was March of 2019. We did multiple tests. My doctor sent me to three different cardiologists. Every single one looked at me and said if you feel like you're going to faint, sit down. That was the recommendation. No medicines, nothing. Just if you feel like you're faint, you need to sit down. I said to the last one, I would. I do, I have to. He said well, most people won't. I said okay. I thought I'm done, I'm not doing this, I'm just going to keep pushing. My doctor actually called me and said I want to see you again. I went in and I said I'm done. This is ridiculous, I'm not going to continue to do this. He said can you just please see one more cardiologist? I said absolutely. So, I did. It was a female. I had my first appointment with her and she said I looked through your records because I had said to her, they said I had a heart attack, like a mild heart attack, and she said you've had *three* and this is something that we need to take care of immediately. From that point on, it was multiple tests. I don't know all the names of them, I'm not really good at it. I just went and did them and they ultimately pushed and I was in surgery in August of 2021. It did take a little while, but it was more of the cardiologist saying you're fine, you're fine. My doctor kept saying you're not fine, I'm not going to allow this. He kept pushing me to keep going, keep going and keep going, because within that time, I had had several different episodes that I went to the hospital with the same symptoms, same everything. He said this is not normal, you are young, I'm not going to let you not be active and I'm just going to continue to push. So he did. He just kept pushing and pushing for me. When I went to the last cardiologist, she was amazing. She basically said this is bad, this is really bad. People are going to tell you that you don't need to get it fixed. But that's not even an option. I didn't realize it. This is how silly I was.

When they said that I had to have surgery, I thought, oh, it's just going to be really quick, like probably laparoscopic, just get in there and pull that. No, not the case, no joke. A week before I had my pre-op, I go down and it's a doctor from Kaiser, one of our local healthcare systems. He works with some of the Stanford doctors. I had to go for my pre-op and the nurse was telling us this is what we do, this is your process. He said do you have any questions for me? I said, so because you don't have to do like full, full heart surgery, it's probably pretty quick recovery? My mind was like, oh, they're just doing a little "sweater cut" is what he called it. I'm thinking like a sweater cut and the nurse looks at me and said there's no such thing as small heart surgery. "You're having open-heart surgery, Sarah." I asked, like cutting my bone and everything? He said, yes, they had already told me, but I think you just shut it out, like there's no way I have to have full on open-heart surgery. So that was, for me, oh my gosh, this is really serious. But I just have a way of saying it's fine, it's fine, we'll get through it.

Mine was worse when they got in. Initially they said it's a very slight dip into your heart muscle. Once they got in, the surgeon came in afterwards and said, "Had you not gotten this done, the next time I would have seen you, you would not have been alive." It had been not enough that they had to do a bypass. They were thinking they might have had to take an artery from another part of my body and put it in. He said it was way deeper than we thought and it was definitely deteriorating. Mine went really quick. It sounds like yours was the same thing, Jeff. Right?

JH: Yes. Similar.

Sarah Miller: I went from running five miles at a certain pace to where I couldn't even run three steps without my heart rate getting to 220. I could still move and do things. I was just exhausted. Mine was more about being tired than it was like I couldn't breathe. I could do all of that. If I got super active, my whole left side would go numb, my neck, my jaw, I would feel like I was going to throw up. I could continue to do it. I wasn't so exhausted where, like some people can't. Sounds like you couldn't even walk from one place to another, Veronica.

Veronica Thaxton: No, and you know it just, oh gosh, it hurts me to hear how long you suffered with that from 2013 to 2019. Six years. But I can also relate to that. I was a little more severe when it hit me. It hit me and I declined rapidly and wasn't able to do much of anything. But I can so relate to if you can still get through the rest of your daily activities and you can do, you know, you're just a little more limited when you're pushing yourself. I can totally see this taking forever to finally get something done. It's like, well, I'm pretty fine most of the time.

Sarah Miller: When I'm not, I'm not, but when I'm okay, I'm okay.

Veronica Thaxton: Thank goodness you had that doctor who was willing to push you and say, no, we're not stopping, there's something wrong. I think that's amazing. You've got a really good one. That's great.

Sarah Miller: Once I finally got over the fact that I had to get my chest bone cut I had no nervousness. My family was really nervous about me because they thought are you just not understanding what's happening? I said, no, I'm going to actually feel better. No, I have no nervousness about it, I'm excited. I'm excited to get through it. Then I started realizing, oh, all those symptoms, I'm tired all the time. I would fight it because I didn't like to be tired. I would just say I'm not tired, mind over matter. Not tired all of the time when I was running and struggling to keep up, knowing that, wait, it's not just my cardio, it's not my physical body. Something is not right. But yeah, I didn't notice all of that until afterward.

JH: There is a word for that. It's called denial. I had it massively. None of us want to accept it. It's still hard for me to say I had a heart attack. How do you have a heart attack when you're in great shape? You think you're in great shape and to both of your points if, just on the front side of this discussion, before we get into the post-surgery side, the biggest thing somebody can do is don't think there's nothing wrong, don't deny yourself there's an issue here, because very similar to both of you, I did the same thing. I'm 20 plus years older than both of you. I have the occlusion where the artery enters into the heart. I'll repeat again for anybody that didn't hear Dr. Schnittger's interview, 100%, 100%. Everybody who has a myocardial bridge has plaque buildup where the artery enters the heart. The longer you go with the bridge, the more plaque buildup you're likely going to have. The more plaque, the less blood flow. The less blood flow, the more likely you are to have some sort of a heart issue. I attribute it to the fact, in my case, that I was in pretty good shape all the way up until I wasn't, and my body said, "You're done." You're not going to have a whole lot of time with this, and it was, really rapid deterioration as well. Mine didn't occur under stress as much as it did when not stressed. It worked better, hurt less when I was stressing it.

Sarah Miller: Completely different than mine, until I couldn't, and then everything went to heck and nothing worked.

JH: You both said it. You keep pushing, saying okay, no, there's something not right here. I have to figure this out. You have to advocate for yourself because the doctors don't know, and I do believe the best doctors assume is that it's not to just fix us, it's to get us back to where we were or the best lifestyle they can get for us, not just an acceptance of a bad situation that you saw, Veronica, where, well, that's as good as it's going to get. You're going to be either on meds or just not going to walk around anymore.

Veronica Thaxton: Yes, I did, and I'll have to say I'm with that same cardiologist today and I will see him for my follow-up. My first follow-up is tomorrow. When I said he told me that and I just I know he saw me in the hospital bed shaking my head, saying no, just not accepting that. He said, well, give me a few weeks. Man, he just really turned around and those few weeks he did his research. He found all the Stanford stuff, obviously because he was talking about some of that research and at least did something. He was willing to listen enough to me and to see my non-acceptance of his response and take some action, at least try to get me to Mayo and did more research. Then, when I had these all these great options, I heard back from Chicago, Stanford, Mayo and I set up some time to talk to him about all these options that I had and he had done so much research.

He had talked to a group of other congenital heart disease cardiologists. He texts and they share cases and ask questions. After doing his research, he bounced it off them and they all said Stanford's the place to be and he's a believer now and I think that's a great doctor who is willing to say, okay, maybe there is more to this. I've always thought this was benign, but I see you're not, I'm going to try to help you. Then, to keep researching and see all the literature that's out there and all the case studies and turn around and come up to where we are. It's great. I'm thrilled that I've got a cardiologist in town who can continue to care for me and knowing the before and after. I'm happy to be with him. If there are any other bridge patients hey, here's another case now. He's had one or two or however many, but I'm happy that I ended up with someone who, in the end, was willing to give it another shot or learn more or not accept my "no".

JH: Look at the education we're providing, not only for the cardiologist or the doctors who are getting to work on us, but also for the benefit of everybody else who comes after us as well, now that a cardiologist or surgeon goes, "I get it. I've seen this before. Yeah, it's real. I hear what you're saying because I've heard it before now and I've seen the transfer from symptom to improvement." That's such a big deal. It's the same with my cardiologist, who was open to saying "I don't know what's wrong with you. We need to find somebody who can help figure it out." Sarah, it sounds like you found the female cardiologist who said you're right, something's wrong here.

Sarah Miller: Yeah, it was no question to her. She said I got your file and I thought why hasn't something already been done and why are you saying you have not had a heart attack and why are they okay with that? It was interesting. I step back and think I have sent my records out. You were also very persistent with yours; my doctor was persistent with me. I mean, obviously they tell me I'm going to have open-heart surgery and I don't even I know what it is.

My doctor advocated for me from that point on, and I'm very, very fortunate because I don't know if I would have done that for myself until it was too late, which is sad, but it's hard to admit, it's hard to say this is what it is. I also have another condition that I was born with, hypertrophic cardiomyopathy. (hardening or thickening of the heart muscle) Mine's at the tip of my heart and they don't think when they went in to do surgery, they don't think that was part of the problem. They looked at it and said I think we're good. They did some tests when they were in there, said they might have to do more surgery if they felt like it was bad. They were able to do a function type of test to see.

I guess technically, it's a part of my heart that's dead, that was not effective. That also scared her when she saw that as well. She actually was the one that found that. She found that because she ordered an MRI of my heart and some special MRI that showed angles that would not typically show or be shaded, she was so thorough. I'm indebted to her and my actual primary care doctor because they were the ones that said this is not okay and anybody who has said anything up to this point, we are disappointed.

JH: Let's transition now from what got us to our surgery to where we are today. Veronica, you were the catalyst for this conversation because I knew you were so early on when we talked. I have a friend who's a cardiac nurse at the hospital system here in Sacramento and she mentions she knows this guy, one of her good friends has this thing called a myocardial bridge to one of her friends on the floor and she goes hey, I have a friend that has one of those things too. My friend, the nurse, calls and she goes, "Jeff, you're not going to believe this, somebody else has your condition and they live in the Sacramento area. They're in Folsom, California," which is 10 minutes from my house. I'm blown away. That's awesome! I asked, do you think you could ask her, knowing HIPAA (Health Insurance Portability and Accountability Act, which governs patient privacy), would you please ask your nurse friend if she would ask her friend, if I can call her just so I can figure out what the heck is going on? And, sure enough, the person happened to be Sarah. Our first phone call, she spent over an hour, it was a Sunday afternoon and she talked with me for an hour about oh, this is this and this is that and she's already a year out of it. I'm not in it yet and I'm thinking, oh God, this is going to be rough because how long until I can ride again? She had already started running by then too, so we had this wonderful conversation and have since maintained a relationship. If you would go now to your next step, you get your surgery date. You're going to Stanford. It's not like you're going to Northern California for vacation, even though you pack the bag and you're excited. It's a little bit different. And now it's time, this is less than seven weeks ago. What has been happening since and walk us through post-surgery.

Veronica Thaxton: Yeah, so when I packed my bags for those three weeks, California wasn't quite this spa vacation.

JH: Right.

Veronica Thaxton: But, man, it was the next best thing. The care that I received was world-class. I went up there for the week of testing and the surgery, the unroofing followed by a modified Ravitch procedure. And you know, Jeff, I'm just still so thankful to you because you know we hear what the surgery is, or from what the recovery is like from a sternotomy. But I had no idea what to expect with modified Ravitch recovery, and so I couldn't prepare myself before. When I got home and I was feeling terrible, I reached out to you and sent a message and said hey, you're the only one I know who also had the same situation, when do you feel better? I think that was the gist of the message because, man, I was struggling.

JH: Let me just add, for the people who don't know what this modified Ravitch procedure that Veronica is talking about is. We have the sternotomy, so we're like most others who have the sternum cut down the center and then the surgeon in our case happened to be the same surgeon. Dr Boyd finishes up and he pins that back together as it would be closed, and then the thoracic surgeon comes in because our sternums are deeper into our chest, causing pressure on our hearts, at least in my case. I'm assuming it'll be something similar to yours too. They don't want to do all this work on the heart and then still find out that the sternum is putting pressure on the heart. They have to lift the sternum, and that's what the modified Ravitch procedure is. It requires cutting ribs from the sternum. So not only do you have the healing process of the incision from the sternotomy, now you have ribs that have to grow back to the sternum that's been adjusted in some way, shape or form to relieve the pressure on the heart. Yeah, it's just a little more fun in the healing process. As a functional process, it heals at the same time.

It's still roughly a 12-week process, and I remember talking to Dr. Boyd about it. I said, okay, Dr. Boyd, we're going to do all this and he goes you're going to get your buddy, Dr. Berry, and he's going to come in and we're going to do all this stuff. I said, then what? Well, yours is going to be a little different. It's going to be a little more painful. I'm thinking you don't really want somebody to tell you this is going to hurt more, because all you can think about is more is relative on a scale. What does more mean?

You're still in that space a little bit. For those of you learning this—those who are going to have this extra process—the symptoms you'll experience will still be similar.

So you go through your surgery, you get to ICU.

Veronica Thaxton: Yes, you're right. It's true that there's a little more pain. I've never had a sternotomy so I can't compare, but apparently, it's true that there's a little more pain when the modified Ravitch is involved. I got a little bonus time. I didn't get out of there until Saturday night from the Thursday morning surgery and my blood pressure is just normally a little bit low. I was having a little bit of trouble with that, trouble keeping oxygen up and pain control. Goodness, it was just a real feat for them to be able to get on top of pain and nausea. So, I had a little extra time in ICU but great care while I was there. And you know, I don't want to scare anyone away from surgery, make anyone nervous about the pain, because I think everyone who's had this says it's painful. It's rough. But you can do it and that's so true. It's just going to be rough for a little bit. They take great care of you. They do everything they can to help you and it's just something you have to get through and you do make it.

When I reached out to you, Jeff, about three weeks post-op, and said when does this get better? You said it will, and it does. Dr. Schnittger told me in my follow-up at one week that typically with the unroofing that people start feeling better. At week three to four post-op, she said you're going to feel bad for six weeks and I said okay, and that was true. It was six weeks last Thursday and yesterday was the first day I woke up and thought I feel good and today. I feel like myself and it's the first time since August of 2021 that I have felt like myself.

After surgery it's tough, it's inconvenient, you know you're limited in your range of motion and just getting along. I had a great support system. I had friends and family come up to Palo Alto. I had lots of support at home.

That was a great help. Other than that, it's just getting through. I know that I do want to mention, I think we hear a lot of people worry about ICU and worry about waking up from surgery intubated and they dread it. I have to say, don't be scared. I was very prepared. I was somewhat like you, Sarah, I was never nervous about surgery, I was never scared, always ready, always excited. When you know that there's a possibility that you could wake up intubated, it's the pain. You say, okay, well, I know that it could be there and you deal with it, and I woke up intubated for a couple hours. It's a little uncomfortable, but it's not the only thing you've got going on and they keep you comfortable and it's just not something to worry about.

Sarah Miller: I think we want to tell people what it feels like to be in pain. Tell people what it feels like because I didn't have anybody. I don't know anybody. I didn't have a group. I just shut it out and thought I'm going to deal with it because I don't know even what to expect. I didn't have the extra element of your surgeries. I think that probably alleviated a lot of my pain because I didn't have that. I don't want to surprise anybody, but I would be so thankful to hear somebody say this is the amount of pain and this is how long. Then you have something to grasp. I just dealt with it and I was really fortunate. I didn't have a lot of pain. I had a really, really bad headache and I had back pain. I don't know if either one of you had back pain.

JH: Oh yeah, we talked about that.

Sarah Miller: When I got out, my pain went away in about two weeks. I think it was so painful that you also forget. When I talked to Jeff the other day, I'm like, okay, I have to figure out how much pain. You forget about it. It's been a year-and-a-half now, but I started thinking about it over the next couple of days and thought, yeah, for the first two weeks. Then I talked to my husband, how much pain was I really in? Because I will pretend like I wasn't in as much pain. He reminded me I was in a lot of pain, but two weeks for me. I was also told that that you could have the surgery and not have that extreme bone pain. Some people could have even more extreme bone pain. Yeah, it is painful in all sorts and everyone's going to have their own things. I had a really, really hard time, probably about six months after, where I would have this intense pain. I think it was muscle spasming where you felt like you were going to throw up. I could not focus. I couldn't do anything. I was taking so much Advil and anything I could get my hands on. I don't take that typically. I didn't grow up with medicines. I couldn't even bear it. I absolutely could not bear the pain, but it went away. It was muscle spasms. I don't think everyone even gets those though.

JH: I'm going to refresh your memory, Veronica, as we talk about pain management, because it is significant, and the hospital is the first one to say we want to manage the pain. We want you to be able to do things and not do them because of the pain. They give us a regimen of what we can tolerate and I know the three of us here don't want to tolerate any meds. For anybody who tolerates an opioid or whatever the drug they give you, take it, because it is important. There's a reason for that. Veronica was talking to me when I called her and she said well, I stopped everything because I thought I just didn't want to take the drugs. I didn't want to take the Tylenol, and two days later, after everything had cleared your system, you were in excruciating pain, if I'm not mistaken.

Veronica Thaxton: I took some Tylenol. When they released me looking back on it, Jeff, it's just ridiculous. I mean they couldn't manage my pain in the hospital. So I'm released and I don't take the pain meds other than Tylenol, and then wonder why I can't walk more than you know 10 or 15 steps and I was in a lot of pain. It doesn't just mean while you're here under our care in the hospital, take the pain meds, it means when you get out and Sarah, I'm the same, I have a high tolerance to pain. I thought I can handle this, I can push through it. We push through so much pain and you ignore it and you just grit your teeth and you go, and I kept doing that. But I was so limited. And what happens is, my lungs aren't healing as well as they should, because my activity isn't where it should be and I'm just in pain. My checkup with Dr. Boyd, when I'm telling him how far I can walk, they're like oh no, you should be walking five or 10 minutes this week and 10 to 15 minutes next week. I'm like, no, we're talking steps, not minutes for me. So they got me back on the pain schedule. You need to take this painkiller and then, three hours later, you need to take the ibuprofen. Getting back on that schedule, I was able to function, which you need to do. It's so important. I think we think we're tough and we can handle pain, and we can to a certain extent. But can we enough that our bodies are really allowed to heal? If I'm gritting my teeth on the couch, getting through the pain, but I'm not moving, my lungs aren't re-inflating, then what am I really doing to help along my recovery? That was a whole mindset that I had to realize I needed to adopt, and I did that the hard way. I did have to get back on the pain meds. That's a little while, and you know they're not fun. I don't feel great on them. I feel a little woozy, a little nauseated, but you know you need it and you will eventually come off. It's okay to be on them and it's okay to let your body heal and you're going to come off. It's not forever.

Sarah Miller: You were on heavier meds because of the extra surgical work.

JH: Yes. And everybody's pain is different, so the necessity for the medication really is going to be predicated on the intensity of the pain. In my case I was off the opioids in two days, but I couldn't eat enough Tylenol. It was every four hours. I don't recall the dosage. I don't even want to say the dosage because I don't want to imply that's acceptable, but it was as much as they said you can tolerate and do it every four hours. And I did that, initially it was a little rough, but the pain was manageable. Then, it started to minimize and minimize and minimize. Opioids just screw my entire system up. I said I'm going to do everything I can to not have to take that if I don't have to. It was just a couple of days, but that Tylenol was another six weeks, eight weeks, and then, as you finally get to start cutting it back which you do, Veronica, you're correct, it's exciting. You wake up and you tell your wife hey, I only had to take, you know, x number of pills today and I can't wait until I'm only doing it twice a day and pretty soon, I won't be taking them at all. I want that to be great. There was another thing that happens with the pain too that I think we forget, and I want to bring it up because I know I talked to you about it. We all experienced this crazy back pain. I couldn't find a solution to it. I went and bought a heating pad right away and I laid on it and I think I shared with you, Veronica, I built this rig on the couch that had variations of the day as the day would go on. I would sit against the rig so that I could have the heating pad in the right spot and move it around, and then I would go to bed and it would hurt like heck and I thought, well, why don't I just take the heating pad to bed? That'll make all the difference in the world, and it did until I didn't need it any longer. You do have to experiment around, you have to move and find places you can sit and get comfortable to where you're upright, not laying down all the time, because that's not good either.

Sarah Miller: I got physical therapy really early on. I have a really good friend who owns the practice. It was super gentle, like she knew how to work it. That was a game changer for me because it was yeah, when I woke up and I see you, I said to the nurse he was the best guy ever. Oh, my gosh, he was amazing, he was my angel. I wasn't in so much pain; I had the worst headache. I said to him I don't know what is going on with my back and my shoulder. He said do you want me to show you what they did when you were in surgery? I said yeah, and he said no, really, do you want to really see? He showed me the way that they have to position you and he said this is exactly why you feel this way. It was a good visual for me, because you think, oh, it's going to hurt here, not my whole body, so it took a long time. My collar bones are still kind of a little wonky and I have to go back to my PT. She helps rearrange it a little bit and I have a masseuse who also does it as well, but it'll never be straight again. Which is fine with me, I'm okay with that. I can run. Small trade off.

Veronica Thaxton: You know, both those things, still sore at the collar bone and went today for the first time and got a guy I go to for active release treatments and he was able to work the intercostals back inside of those ribs and just really help gently, loosen things up again. Even six weeks out ribs are still out of whack. But that made a huge difference.

Sarah Miller: Yeah. I don't know if I ever asked this of you, Jeff, when you breathe. I'm assuming that is even more painful because you actually had ribs that were cut.

JH: Oh, yeah, breathing. They give you the little spirometer and they tell you you're getting out and now do this thing you know, three, four times a day and I'm going to be religious about it because I want to be able to breathe. It hurts like hell to take a deep breath, especially if you're trying to minimize the pain meds. Then you have to blow it out hard and then draw it into the spirometer and that hurts like hell, but you get used to it. Again, that's very critical. It really is. For anybody who's recovering from the surgery, the spirometer is important because it gives your lungs the volume and you need that. I said, well, if all that's been cut and moved around and opened up, maybe I can get more air in there now because it's a little loose. So I'm going to take these big, big, deep breaths and push really, really hard and push it all out. I don't know if it made any difference, but it was a good idea at least in my mind.

Sarah Miller: I was thinking I'm going to get more. This is going to help my running. I thought I was thinking too hard.

Veronica Thaxton: Same here, Sarah, you're going to be so fast.

Sarah Miller: You know how the nurse comes to your house for two weeks after. Did you have this?

JH: No, did you, Veronica? I had no nurse come to my house.

Sarah Miller: No? It was supposed to be four weeks that they would come and check up on me once a week and check to make sure I'm doing my thing. I also was religious. I did it when I was supposed to do it. I did my walks four times a day. God, they told me I could go to here. I went to there and pushed it a teensy bit enough to not be bad. But the nurse who came to the house said this was very shocking. I just thought you just got open heart surgery. I'm doing everything I'm supposed to be doing. I was talking to him. He was young. He said he just went and visited somebody else who had open heart surgery. They got to their house and they were drinking soda and playing video games and had not touched anything. Nothing, wow, nothing. And I thought how precious our life is. How do you not do a simple thing because it's painful and it's scary? When you know it's time to do the thing, darn it. I don't want to do the thing.

He basically said to this person we're not coming to you because we want to come to people like you, meaning me. You know how important it is. You're doing the things that you're supposed to be doing and when you do that, you are going to come out of it a lot better. And even though I don't know necessarily what they said to you, Veronica, my surgeon was very honest. He said we're going to fix you but you won't be able to do the same things as you did prior. That's hard and I know you and I have talked about that and you have to change. That mindset of your level is here and you're still going to be able to go back and do it. It just may not look the same. I struggled with that on my first training for my marathon. It was so hard to mentally have to not do what you did before until I did the marathon and I thought I got to do this again. Who cares what the time is, I get to do it. I get to wake up every single morning and I get to run and do the things that I love and I'm not tired like I used to be. I'm not. That was huge for me to just have to step back and say, okay, this is my new me and that's okay because you're an athlete. I don't know what yours said to you, but it was good that my surgeon said to me we're going to make it a lot better. Just know that it may not be the same as when you were at your height.

Veronica Thaxton: You know, Dr. Boyd said send me a picture of your next triathlon. He said that I would be able to get back to it, but he didn't really set any expectations for me. He didn't say you're going to be able to do it, but watch out for this, or know that you'll be at half your performance level or 75%. I don't know that yet. I guess I'll see what I'm able to do. But for you, Sarah, what was your return to training like? How did you approach it? When did you start and how did you increase your efforts?

Sarah Miller: I got to start running at 12 weeks and my friend, who's a PT, is also a runner and specializes in recovery. I giggled for two reasons. I giggled when I saw it because I thought, oh my gosh, this is really simple. And then I giggled because I went, I don't even know if I could do it. I think I did like a one-minute then three-minute walk and then I could do three minutes, and then it just built on itself. It was a 12-week program. It took me 12 weeks to get back to running three straight miles and I had to keep my heart rate under a certain number, so I would have to slow down to keep it under. 12 weeks. Then I started marathon training. At that point marathon training at three miles was my long run on a Saturday. Other than, like normally, we would jump out and do 10 or something to be our base.

Veronica Thaxton: Little different.

Sarah Miller: And those three miles were not pretty. I was not a nice person and thankfully my best friend who runs with me, bore with me because it was really humbling to me. I thought, oh, this is why people maybe don't like running. It's really hard, it's really hard.

Veronica Thaxton: Were the new limitations self-imposed or was it because of the surgery? Did you say, okay, I need to keep it at this pace or HR under this level.

Sarah Miller: The first 12 weeks he said I can't have it go over a certain amount. Then I went back and they said, okay, you're good to do whatever you want to do. Then the fear set in for me. That's when I started having a lot of fear and I think that probably still holds me back. I just don't push like I have pushed before because it's scary and I think if I could just stay here, I'm fine, I just want to run. We were talking earlier that I did a 50-miler. I am out there smiling the entire time because I think I get to do this. Still, I'm not going to push it because I'm not going to ruin this and the ability to do it. They actually said to me initially, you can't do anything over 26 miles. I said OK. Then my friend asked me if I wanted to do the American River 50-miler and I said, well, let me ask my doctor and let me ask my surgeon. I did and I was very honest with them. I said here's what I want. This is what I've been doing. Am I okay to do it? And they said as long as you smile and you breathe, we will let you do it, but you're never going over 50. I'm like, okay, I won't to do that anymore.

I now go into those events with a very different mindset. I'm just so happy that I get to be here, that I am not willing to push it and test the limits anymore, which I used to, and you have to set your ego aside and let people pass you. My time wasn't exactly what I wanted, but it's because I didn't push myself and I'm okay with that now. Prior, had I not pushed myself hard enough, I would have been upset at myself. It's fun. It makes it a little bit more fun to just go out with no expectations. Just finish. You just get to finish.

Veronica Thaxton: And enjoy it and taking the pressure off yourself. That's great.

Sarah Miller: And actually experience what's around you. I would never stop at a station, ever, never stopped at aid stations. I wouldn't have my phone out, I wouldn't look at people. I was just going forward, that's it. Now I'm like, oh my gosh, I saw a bald eagle. I really did on my run. I stopped; I took a picture of it. It was just a different lens of what I used to see. I'm really, really, really happy about it.

JH: If I were your therapist, I'd tell you," You've come a long way."

Sarah Miller: I have.

Veronica Thaxton: So happy to hear that. I have some angry moments in my house.

Sarah Miller: I will be honest. I screamed because I thought this is what life is, this is what it's going to be right after four weeks. You still can't lift five pounds. I had a couple of moments my husband had to calm me down and remind me that I just had surgery. But I'm like, I can do it. And he said, you can't right now, you have to wait.

JH: I think one of the things you'll find as well, Veronica, your six-and-a-half weeks, let's say even at 12, that's where I was cleared to get on the bike, on a trainer in the garage and they said, it's okay, you could ride, but what if you fell? Then you're going to make a mess of all the work we just did and I said, oh, ok, well, that makes sense, because I think I can ride. It's not about the ride, it's not about the heart, it's about the damage you could do if you fell on the bike. I'm a year almost to the day. Last year at this time when I first got on the trainer in the garage and they said, give us another month before you go out on the bike. Getting on the trainer, I was so excited. I had my wife video it and you know, I'd thanked everybody for the ability for me to even be able to get back on it.

I cried when I started pedaling and I cried when I got off it, thinking I get to do this again. I get to do this again and I know I can get off the trainer at some point. Everything worked and I had no symptoms. The only thing that was really unusual is the discomfort came from the pressure on the healing bone. All the sternum area that has had all the work and part of my modified Ravitch included a bar that stayed in there for a year. I would feel that discomfort. You're holding the handlebars and you're close and you've got your body weight on it. So that was there. I felt that. I wouldn't call it pain but discomfort more than anything.

And that first ride four weeks later, on the street, I'm going out on the bike and I'm clipping into pedals and I'm thinking what if I can't get my leg down. What if I fall? All of it worked out just fine. That healing process, all of it, it does take time and just because the 12 weeks is where you can pick things up, it doesn't mean it's okay. It's not all done. It really takes at least a year for all of that to heal properly and do everything that it's supposed to do. I was fortunate I got back in the gym as well. I got back in the gym in June, so I waited six months and started with extremely, extremely light weights again. Talk about humbling. Humbling when you know what you used to do. Here you are with these baby weights. But it does improve and I know we might be talking over a lot of people who don't exercise the way we do, but it's scalable. It's the same as it is for somebody who is more sedentary. Just get up and walk around the block. That is a big deal for some people and all of our doctors will tell us, have told us and probably tell every other patient, that your well-being is related to all of your body—and to your mind to a greater degree. You feel better by doing something and you're not going to heal well if you don't. You're at six-and-a-half weeks and you look and sound remarkable. I don't know that I looked and felt like that at six and a half weeks.

Sarah Miller: You actually said something so important though, Jeff. It's the mental part. They also prepped me for that, because I think we think with our type of brains, it's not going to affect us. It does. And I think we're all really strong mentally. But I started meditating because I thought I'm not going to get hit with the depression. I simply don't want to. I did research on it because, especially with the heart, there is a huge connection. I was more afraid of that than I was of the pain, I think. I started meditating, started journaling, even prior to surgery because I wanted to make sure that was not a part that I fell deep into. Because you're in pain, you weren't moving, just sitting and then you start going down this dark, dark place and it's hard to come back from that. It's super important for people to make sure that they are aware when they start feeling that way. Another thing is my doctor said a lot of times when people start feeling hopeless and felt lost, it's actually a physical issue that we don't know. He said if you start feeling helpless or really depressed, you need to come back in because that could be potentially something going wrong with your surgery. I thought, interesting, I wouldn't have thought of that, I would have just thought I'm not moving, I don't get to do what I normally do. I have a strong personality. But it is really important that if you start feeling that hopeless, feeling that what is this life worth, check in with your doctor quickly.

Veronica Thaxton: I had read about this impact. I began going to yoga five to seven days a week. I guess the beginning in January 2022 because I just couldn't work out, I couldn't do anything but the yoga. Really, it's like an hour-long stretching class. I couldn't hold any body weight, it's none of the typical warrior poses or anything. It was yen yoga, an hour-long stretching, but the beginning has meditation and that really helped mentally prepare me as well.

Sarah, I think what you're saying makes sense. You need to prepare yourself for it. Then, reading about some of the mental and emotional aspects that you can encounter after surgery, I wanted to be prepared for that too. You know where I found that it helped me most was in leading up to surgery. Some of the frustration that I had, was coming from such an active lifestyle to just sitting on the couch. I spent as much time sitting on the couch pre-surgery as I did post-surgery, just because my activities were so limited, it really helped me get through that. It helps me in the testing. It helped me get through testing. When you wake up intubated, you're just totally chill because you can be. You've learned to relax, you've learned how to work through things and be patient. As far as any other pre-or post-counseling or discussions about hey, this could pop up, no, I didn't really have any, so

I'll be looking forward to your podcast that focuses on that. I think that's such an important aspect people need to think about.

JH: People do experience it and they may think it's just them. It's not just them, it's many. When so many things in your life change and you realize your mortality, that's a big deal and you have a constant reminder because something hurts. You're there with that frustration or pain for quite some time. It wears on you after a while. Meds aside, you go out to do what you thought you used to be able to do and you can't do any of it. Strike two. Then you go and you get a little bit better, and you go to do what you think you could do because that's what you used to do before. I can't do that now and it just piles on. I think the awareness and recognition of the gift we've been given to get up every day again as a result of the surgery is simply amazing. Everybody I talked to who is symptomatic, we all have this concern that we don't know if you could die, and you just don't know if this thing's going to kill you. If it is, when? We never get to know the termination point. At least now, we know we've been given this gift for a reason, what do we do with it and how do we do things differently and still enjoy the stuff that we did before? That helps us be stronger.

So you did your run. I have to share this because I want to give Veronica some encouragement here. I did my first organized ride on Saturday as well, and it was 65 miles in the Sierras. It was spectacular. The whole time I'm thinking, okay, this is not a race, it's not competitive. Just watch your heart rate. Dr. Boyd just said don't overdo it and I had been training for it. I felt really, really good and it was everything I could do to intentionally moderate and not be stupid. Even though I felt I could be stupid, everything felt good. But what a gift. A year ago and pre-surgery, no way. So you're just back to that recovery process. The funny thing is, you forget it. You forget the intensity and the duration and the frustration of the pain and we get to the end and I pulled over and I just sat on the back of the car and cried. I couldn't have done this before. You know I'm so fortunate and so blessed that I get to do it. In the grand scheme, by all of us being here, we're benefiting somebody else who gets to see that this is a condition that is treatable, it does improve, not necessarily the same for everybody, but it does.

Veronica Thaxton: Congratulations on the great ride. What a milestone. I can imagine how that must have felt when you finished.

JH: I remember when I asked Dr. Boyd how many people didn't make it off the table after the surgery and he looks at me and goes "none." *Everybody* made it off the table. Not everybody made it long term, but some of that was by choice and some of it was by complications, other conditions, and he said I don't have any expectation for anybody that does what they're supposed to do that they shouldn't be able to live a healthy life as a result. I hope we're providing some of that incentive for the other people too.

Veronica Thaxton: I'm glad to share my journey for anyone who has questions further down the road. I appreciate both of you sharing your journeys with me. It's helped me tremendously and I just appreciate that the myocardial bridge Facebook group is also full of great responses.

JED BAKER:
A Bridge Too Far

(A clinical psychologist knows, he's not just imagining his symptoms.)

We are about to explore Jed's challenging journey through the maze of medical uncertainty and misdiagnosis, highlighting the silent battles his heart endured. Jed's story is a testament to resilience, showcasing the human spirit's ability to persevere amidst elusive medical conditions. His journey began with sudden symptoms, such as shortness of breath and dizziness, leading to multiple inconclusive tests and a frustrating cycle of uncertainty.

The turning point came with the discovery of a myocardial bridge, revealed after an emergency catheterization, emphasizing the need for thorough cardiac evaluations when initial tests fall short.

Jed's narrative is enriched by his bond with Kaylin Kellert and Leanne Aigner, his "surgery sisters," who shared similar surgical journeys and dates. (Their stories can be heard on the "Imperfect Heart" podcast.) Their experiences underscore the impact of community and support during difficult times. Together, they navigated the complexities of cardiac care, exploring treatments and ultimately opting for unroofing procedures. This chapter highlights the importance of second opinions and the courage needed to advocate for one's health. Jed's story offers a broader commentary on facing health challenges, emphasizing informed decision-making, emotional resilience, and hope. It serves as a cautionary tale and hope for anyone dealing with similar medical mysteries, illustrating that perseverance and community can guide the path to recovery.

Jed Baker (Guest): Jeff, I've listened to your voice so many times, that comforting voice of yours, and you're like a ray of hope in pretty dark times for some of us who've been going through this, it's been a wonderful opportunity that you have me here and I get to see and hear you in person.

Jeff Holden (Host): Jed, I'm humbled by that coming from somebody of your pedigree and…

Jed Baker: Pedigree, pedigree! That and my E-Z pass get me through the tolls on the New Jersey turnpike.

JH: No pedigree?! I'm talking to an author and a clinical psychologist who is complimenting me on my voice. You talk to people all day long to calm them down and get them on the right track, thank you for that.

We're going to have an interesting conversation because you have gone through your process, concurrent with a couple of other people that we had on the program and that would be Kaylin Kellert and Leanne Aigner, all in the same 24-hour period, you're the triumvirate of surgery here.

Jed Baker: They're my surgery sisters and I watch out for everything they say. I've been feeling like I've been in it together with them from the get-go.

JH: In a bit of irony, the three of you going through the process at the same time is really unique. There are not that many surgeries being done in the course of a week, much less to have two of you at one place and a third on the other side of the country, when we're all trying to find the proper surgeon and the proper diagnosis.

You're 59 years old, obviously had this all your life. As we know, it's a birth defect, but it wasn't until relatively recently that you started to experience symptoms. Walk us through when that occurred and what the symptoms were that you were experiencing.

Jed Baker: Sure, I think my story, symptom-wise, begins four to five years ago. It was just before COVID. I had some kind of wacky virus and I never really run a fever. I had a fever that lasted a day. I recovered.

I'm always well and then one day I woke up in the middle of the night gasping for air, couldn't breathe well and I felt really dizzy and I'm looking to my wife and my daughter was in the house. Something's not right. They took me to the emergency room, I was still trying to catch my breath there, they gave me some oxygen and such and I guess they did some sort of routine tests. They do your labs to see if you've had a heart attack, which fortunately I didn't. They do the EKG, which you know. By the time I got there it was sort of normal again, and so that was my first ER visit where, like a mystery, nobody knows what happened. You seem fine, spend the night, we'll observe you next morning. Leave, go home, okay.

Then I'm at my office, maybe some weeks later, seeing clients and I would get bloated and couldn't breathe. I figured, well, this is gastro. Then I got to the point where I'm feeling dizzy again, I can't breathe, drove myself to the ER, which is really not fun when you're dizzy. I get there, and my wife meets me there.

Another round of testing. Maybe they did an echo (cardiogram). I'm not sure what they did, but the third ER visit back in 2019, they did a CT scan which should be able to identify a bridge. As I've learned through this process, only if people are looking for it. I get a CT and they say to me well, you know, Mr. Baker, there's good news and there's bad news, right? The good news is your calcium score is zero. But there's some soft plaque blockage, maybe up to 40%, in your right coronary artery. We don't think that could cause your symptoms but it's enough to put you on a statin.

I started a statin and, by the way, when they finally found my bridge, it was in the LAD (left anterior descending artery). There was nothing in the RCA (right coronary artery). It was clear. Statins work, by the way, because four years later or, as I've also learned, CT scans can be unreliable because it might have been that there really was no soft plaque blockage. At any rate. I go on a statin. They send me back home again and suggest I see my gastro guy. I see a lung person. Why can't I breathe? Right? This is a little different than I hear from my compadres on the myocardial bridge site.

JH: It seems like you didn't have any vasospasm or endothelial dysfunction. It was more shortness of breath and discomfort?

Jed Baker: Shortness of breath is a scary thing when you don't know that you're going to be able to breathe, and I have to say in retrospect as a kid, growing up, I never felt like I had any symptoms, but I always remembered I'm a great swimmer. I love swimming, but I always had dreams of drowning and not being able to breathe, and I think that's probably at some level I was having a little bit of this occasionally, without knowing it.

Anyway, I go to my gastro guy back in 2019. He says look, maybe you have small intestinal bacterial overgrowth, although they didn't do a test for it. Try this antibiotic, I take the antibiotic. We're now into the pandemic. It's January, nobody's doing anything. We're all hunkered down at home. For whatever reason, my symptoms abated. I just wasn't feeling anything and over the course of four years, on occasion I would get out of breath. I do a lot of speaking engagements for my living and was doing a talk once, I remember, and it was a six-hour talk, so halfway in, and it was after eating for me, I ate lunch, and I go and do this talk, and I remember I'm really having trouble breathing. I told them they could all hear it while I was talking and I said to everybody, don't worry, I'm not having a heart attack. I've been to the ER three times, we know it's nothing.

JH: To the contrary.

Jed Baker: Right. And then I got on a plane to go home and I'm having trouble breathing the whole time on the airplane and I'm bloated too. I'm still thinking it's gastro, which, by the way, I'm sure I have some gastro issues. I might have borderline asthma too, but as the gastro guy and all his office people would say, it shouldn't cause that much shortness of breath. Over the course of four years, it was manageable.

I would feel that the exercise was fine. In fact, I felt better with exercise. Then we hit January 2023, I get COVID and I'm certainly tired after COVID, and then that summer comes around and I'm feeling really tired all the time and I'm looking at my Apple watch and it says you're aerobically not fit anymore and I'm like, really? I would try to push it a little bit and do more exercise. I just kept telling my wife I'm so tired. I went to my primary care doctor. All these tests, everything, lab tests, you're negative. Nothing, nothing's going on. We don't see anything.

JH: For the benefit of those who are wondering what "this tired" is, for those of us experiencing it, it's not tired like, "Oh, I'm a little drowsy. Maybe if I just took a nap." It's complete exhaustion. It's, "I'm done." It's an experience that is not your normal, "I didn't sleep well last night." It's a complete and utter exhaustion type of tired.

Jed Baker: I thought it was old age, right? I said, well, okay, I've reached a certain age. The doctor says no, this is more fatigue than old age, but they couldn't find anything. September, I get my fifth COVID booster, which I handled the other ones fine, but the day after I started to get some palpitations. Now in retrospect I put that together in my head, I may have had little palpitations here and there that I just ignored, but these were certainly bigger. I'm ignoring it. My wife says you should get it checked out, you really should. So I go see the doctor and they put me on a Holter monitor and they see these paroxysmal AFIBs. (Atrial fibrillation) That means it comes and goes, but some of them were an hour and a half long.

They decide well, let's get you another echo. Echo looks great. They said, well, we should just do a stress test to be sure. Meanwhile, I think they're suggesting you don't have to do it now, but you should try a beta blocker if the AFIB continues. I was the type of guy who was getting it only at rest, only after eating, not after exercise, although during this period, for the first time in my life, I started to have some symptoms after exercise. I hadn't had it before. I decided to take a hike up a pretty tall hill by my house and I got to the top and I'm dizzy, I don't feel well and I'm not sure if I can get home. I managed to make it home, but I've not felt that way before. Doc says get the stress test, a *nuclear* stress test. The stress test comes back and the first part they get back is just the EKG part and it looks great. You're not even having any arrhythmia, looking good and I'm like great! I go to the gastro guy because I'm still having some of that bloating and out of breath again here and there. The gastro guy says, well, again, it could be SIBO, small intestinal bacterial overgrowth. We'll start on the antibiotic again. I'm in his office literally talking about this and I get a call from the cardiology office: "The nuclear part of the stress test came back. You have ischemia." I said, "Is it like lack of oxygen to your heart? Is it where you found four years ago that right coronary artery?" "Not at all, it's your anterior, mid-anterior area." Well, that's exactly where the LAD is. I'm ischemic right where the LAD is, I think you're going to need to get a catheterization. Sure, okay, great. So I'm scheduled to get the cath in, I don't know, a week or two. I had already been to the ER twice for shortness of breath in the sequence of time that we've crossed.

Back now in the fall of 2023, I started to get that sort of shortness of breath again. They weren't finding anything. Nothing erratic, no MI, or myocardial infarction.

I was talking to a client on Zoom, not being active, sometimes when you're talking to clients it's emotional. I get irritated and I start to get dizzy and out of breath again and it won't go away. My wife says you've got to go to the ER. I'm saying well, wait, wait, wait. She's not. Let's not mess around. We go to the ER and they say you were scheduled for a week from now, let's do it tomorrow. They do the cath November 10th of 2023. The guy says you have the heart of a teenager. You're great. Incidentally, you have a myocardial bridge in the LAD, mid-LAD area, but it's nothing.

By the way, I'm kind of an obsessive guy as so many of our myocardial bridge compadres are and within about 20 minutes after that diagnosis, I'm thinking, how do I get more information about this? I recalled when my son had a rare issue himself, we found a Facebook site where we found the best surgeons in the country who really know about this. I said maybe there's something like that for myocardial bridges. I look it up, bam, I'm in the myocardial bridge support group. I find out about Stanford. I see that, okay, it's possible one day I might have to have open heart surgery for this. I call the cardiology office, I'm still at the hospital, mind you, and I say to one of his partners, because he's not there hey, I got this myocardial bridge. Could that be causing this issue? He says it's a bridge to nowhere, it's nothing. Don't even bother, don't even worry about it. However, to his credit, my cardiologist comes in about five minutes later and says you know, it's kind of a remarkable finding. He said he's seen the video: "Your artery is getting really constricted. It's getting crushed quite a bit."

JH: He's actually seeing this on the CT, or from the angiogram from the catheterization?

Jed Baker: He's seeing the dye go through the arteries and he's seen it contract and really squeeze on the CT. He's saying it could be something. I said, I've been on this site and it says, it's possible, one day I would need surgery for this. He looks at me and says don't let anybody cut you open. We're going to start with medication. If it doesn't work, we can stent it. I get on the myocardial bridge site. I know how dangerous that is because the bridge, it'll just crush the stent. I get on the myocardial bridge Facebook site, and I say here's what my cardiologist said and, thankfully, all of you guys said WHOA!

JH: You got the flood of information from everyone saying never stent a bridge?

Jed Baker: Yes, and one person who also chimed in was Dr. Kofidis. He says "I don't usually chime in, but this is not a good idea. Don't stent it, and if you want to talk, I'm happy to talk. Not a good idea." I get discharged from the hospital and first thing I do is I listen to your podcast with Dr. Kofidis and learn so much about what's going on, and he's nice enough to have a free Zoom session with me.

JH: Yes, he's very good about that usually within a couple of days.

Jed Baker: Yes. It was no small effort to try to get that cath video from the hospital. I had to really go through hoops just to get a copy of that. Dr. Kofidis said look, take a picture, take a video of it on your phone from your computer screen and send it to me. And he says yes, it's pretty clear. But he says you've got to rule out the gastro stuff again, you've got to rule out the lung things again and you can try medication for three to six months as the protocol is for beta blockers and other things. Do that first, but you clearly have a bridge. It's probably significant.

By the way, the cath that I had was not a provocative cath. There were no flow measurements. Later I asked some folks why, and they said well, we didn't think you had a bridge, so we weren't prepared to do all that, right? But what I have at this point is ischemia right where the bridge is in the same area. I'm not getting oxygen to the heart there, I'm having major SOB, you know shortness of breath symptoms, and I'm having an obvious milking effect. It's clear, right?

I also find out about Stanford's second-opinion program. This is within days, I start sending stuff, and it just takes forever to get the information to them. I was fortunate to get Dr. Schnittger herself to review it, and while I'm waiting for that, I go on the myocardial support page again and find out there's one surgeon in New Jersey who has done at least one unroofing for one person on the myocardial bridge site. I go and see him and he's lovelier than can be. He's just wonderful, spends, I think, an hour-and-a-half with me going over the symptoms. He says look, "I don't think you should be waiting very long for this. You're having significant symptoms, you're ischemic. There's this milking effect. Maybe this needs to get done." It wasn't that hard to find a surgeon.

It turns out in my dense neck of the woods, I have an ER friend who lives in New York City and he knew some heart surgeons. He asked around. He said there's this other guy, Dr. Paul Burns at Valley Hospital which is where I ended up going to meet with him and he was the nicest guy in the world. Like the other guy, I asked both of them how many of these surgeries have you done? The first guy said maybe one a year and he'd been doing this for maybe 10 or 15 years. Dr. Paul Burns, I asked him the same question. He said he's been doing open-heart surgery for 34 years. He said I would say that I have had maybe 10 exclusively unroofing surgeries in my lifetime. However, when I'm doing these bypass surgeries, which he does 400 to 500 a year, very often there's an artery trapped under muscle and he has to unroof it as part of the bypass surgery. He's doing it all the time.

JH: The good news is, just as an aside, we've heard many of the surgeons we've spoken with have the same statement. We've been doing this all along. We just don't consider it an unroofing procedure because they're not symptomatic from what we assume is the bridge. They're symptomatic because the artery is compromised in some way, shape or form. The irony in all that is, according to everybody we've spoken with, 100% of the time where the artery enters the heart, there is compromise. It's either occluded or it's narrowed as a result of the bridge, right?

Jed Baker: Right. And, as I've come to understand as a 59-year-old man, if you stomp on the garden hose for 59 years it may not spring back during diastole again. I'm hoping it springs back. I feel pretty good. I see Dr.

Burns and I think he's great. Here's what really clinched it for me. I went to see another doctor too, head of cardiac surgery at another hospital who has done maybe 20.

By the way, I bet this happens in every state. It certainly happens in New Jersey. The morbidity statistics are calculated for surgeons who do bypass surgery, at least here in the state of New Jersey. I could look up the record of how many of the patients survive for each surgeon at each hospital, by hospital and by surgeon. We're talking about 90-year-old people coming in having a heart attack that they often have to operate on. That's included in those stats. They all had quite good stats. But what clinched it is, while I'm doing these surgery consults and I get Dr. Schnittger's report back, she said look, you definitely have a bridge. It is probably significant. You're ischemic, there's an obvious milking effect and you're having the shortness of breath. It is possible that symptom is responsible for the angina in some people. But our gold standard is that you should have a provocative cath to be sure that the bridge is causing flow problems, blood flow problems. I'm thinking I call one of the surgeons who will do it. Nobody wants to do it here in New Jersey, nobody does. Dr. Paul Burns said I will do it for you, I'll schedule it.

JH: He got the report from Schnittger?

Jed Baker: Yes. He got the report. He not only got the report, but he called me as soon as he got it. The other guy who was great has a zero-mortality rate. He couldn't be bothered to look at the Stanford report. He wanted nothing to do with it. He said, "I've done hundreds more surgeries than I'm sure Stanford has ever done," and you know what, I'm sure he's great and he would have been a competent surgeon, great surgeon. But I needed somebody I also felt I could like and trust to some extent when they're going to open up my chest. Dr. Paul Burns was that guy.

During this period where I'm waiting for the cath again, maybe the provocative cath, I become so out of breath again, I get my third trip to the ER and I call Dr. Burns, his office. He calls me on his cell phone that night. He says "Look, stay there. You did the right thing to go there. You don't have to come to our hospital, stay at the hospital you're at. We'll work this out in the morning. We'll get you the cath. If you like, we'll get you surgery." He says about that provocative cath, "Look, I will do that provocative cath, we can get it scheduled. But you're ischemic, you have obvious milking effect. It's really getting compressed and you're having major symptoms. If you don't meet the cutoff criteria by Stanford University's protocol, what do we do then? Do we say we're not going to do surgery for you? Do we leave you be?"

I failed to mention my trials of beta blockers made my shortness of breath infinitely worse and I felt like I was going to faint, because my blood pressure is always generally low anyway. I felt like I was going to pass out on them. If you have borderline asthma, beta blockers are a bronchial constrictor and can cause more asthmatic-like symptoms. The fact that I now had his cell phone and he's calling me and he's willing to do whatever I want, I said, "You know what, Dr. Burns, I am not up for another procedure. If you think it's inevitable that I'm going to need this unroofing, I'm going to just schedule it." I passed on the provocative cath which I feel mixed about, because maybe it would have shown if I had spasms or I had some endothelial dysfunction. But I was tired and couldn't breathe anymore and I wanted to get unroofed.

JH: Well, there's a level of anxiety when you consider doing this sooner than later. If I wait too long, it may be too late. Am I going to have a heart attack? Am I going to have severe consequences, stroke, whatever it may be. Right? It tends to move you along a little quicker.

Jed Baker: I knew how to prevent having a heart attack. I could sit in a bubble and never move, and that was working. That was working quite well.

JH: At some point in time, though, we do know it will catch up to you, because bridges don't get better. To your point of the compression of the artery over 59 years, 65 years, others 70, it becomes less responsive and rebounds slower and you still have something happening in terms of its narrowing at the point of entry into the heart. So, yes, you would debilitate yourself.

Jed Baker: I was going to the ER every couple of weeks and I had stopped living. I wasn't doing talks, I wasn't seeing clients, I wasn't playing music anymore. I wasn't doing anything and I was, frankly, I was agoraphobic. I was afraid to go out of my house and go to the supermarket because I tried that a couple of times and got really out of breath and didn't feel good and not so comfortable driving home, so I didn't want to have another episode somewhere. I stayed literally, sitting on my couch. That's not a life, so, the decision to get surgery was pretty clear.

JH: It's not a way to earn a living either. You can't work; you can't do what you do.

Jed Baker: That's true. Speaking of that, I was hoping originally to go to Stanford because they're doing all the research. As of January 1st, 2024, New Jersey got rid of every single option for self-employed people like me to be insured by a doctor out of state. I thought, well, how much would it cost to go to Stanford? I was ready to do that if I needed to. Also, Stanford said it had an eight-month waiting list. The folks on the support site said that eight-month waiting list is actually 11 months and my life is over right now. I'm not able to do anything. I don't know that I can wait. The next issue was, okay, I'm going to get surgery. They also recommended what's called left atrial appendage closure and pulmonary ablation. Pulmonary vein ablation. I've had some arrhythmias that were going on prior when this all began. The ablation might help with getting rid of AFIB. If you have AFIB, if it recurs, most blood clots that you can get with AFIB will emanate from the left atrial appendage. So this little pouch off the left atrium, if you close it up or you cut it off and you end up getting AFIB again after surgery you're just unlikely to need to be on blood thinners and you're unlikely to get a blood clot. I went to four people. They all said the same thing: We're going to unroof you; pulmonary ablation and we will clip that atrial appendage. Now, they clip it differently, so one person would surgically cut it and staple it. Another person, the doctor I went to, uses something called an Atriclip, which is basically a bobby pin which is in my heart. Yeah, I got a bobby pin in there!

JH: There's excess material that you didn't start with! Lucky you.

Jed Baker: I agonized over that decision more than the unroofing because my symptoms were all based, as far as I could tell, from the bridge. You got to unroof me and maybe the rhythm issues could have been from the bridge, but they could have been independent of that. The ablation made some sense too. Now you want to take a perfectly good part of my heart that didn't seem like it was having any trouble and either cut it off, clip it, cut the blood supply off so that it atrophies. I was reading about it. That was a real agony for me. I have to say Dr. Burns was incredibly patient with me because I must have asked him 20 different times. I sent him journal articles. Look at this article, look at that article. What about that? Is it going to remodel my heart? There was some evidence if you're a kid, that pouch is a larger proportion of your heart than when you're an adult. There was some issue if you already had heart failure, maybe getting rid of that, because it's considered to be an unloading chamber when you're pumping blood, if there's a little overflow of blood, it can go in that pouch. The last thing a surgeon or cardiologist wants is another doctor from a patient who knows how to research and dig and find what he needs to find to ask the questions. It's like I've got you, don't worry, I've got you, well, he's wonderful, he would smile. He would smile and he would respond to those questions. One of the other doctors who, again, he's very competent, he was really tired of my questions. He said, "I think you're overthinking this." I'm electing to have somebody saw me open, retract my ribs, cut into my heart, put a bobby pin on this pouch and kill off a part of my heart and then put radio heat waves to scar around my pulmonary veins that emanate from my heart. To me, I'm not overthinking this. It seems like a big decision.

JH: At this point, you're actually sharing enough information to save some other people all the homework, because they can just say I heard from another gentleman who had the unroofing procedure, who had the same symptoms and the same process that you want to do on me. Give me some more information and you'll save them a lot of extra work.

Jed Baker: I love that description. All four surgeons in New Jersey and Dr. Schnittger said if they're recommending the LAA closure, go ahead and do it. Great. I finally said okay, let's. I can't tell you the relief I had just making the decision because it's not like a broken bone. You've got to set it. The surgeon said, am I absolutely a hundred percent convinced that you won't have shortness of breath again after the surgery? I can't say that for sure, but I think there's a 90 something percent chance it's going to reduce quite a bit given that you're ischemic, given that we see the milking effect. It's so hard to make the decision for many people. That was the worst part of it.

JH: You have your surgery and you now are close to three months out from sternotomy and unroofing. How are you?

Jed Baker: I'm not perfect.

JH: That's what I want you to share.

Jed Baker: I'm nine weeks right now and I didn't have much pain before surgery. I'd say surgery itself was not painful at all. The surgeon has the big work to do. I just get to lie there with some pretty good drugs. After the surgery and sharing this with my surgery sisters, Kaylin and Liann, I was one day ahead of them actually, I could tell them when you get these chest tubes out, man, is that going to be a relief. That first day was pretty tough. I was having a lot of trouble breathing. Chest tubes were in the way.

JH: They're sticking up against your lungs. Every time you take a deep breath, you're getting stabbed in the center of your chest. I remember wondering what the heck? Nobody told me about that.

Jed Baker: Yes, and when those came out, man, I was relieved. At night I would have trouble breathing lying down and so I had to sleep pretty much upright. Five days in the hospital, went home, continued to need to sleep upright, otherwise I would feel like my lungs were drowning like there was a weight on them. I'd say by the fourth week, I felt a lot more functional and I took the walking seriously. They told me you have to walk every day, and I was walking about three miles a day. I still do that, not all at once, although I can walk a couple miles, two miles all at once, pretty well. I feel like I could do more spirometer.

JH: You're working with your spirometer, majorly, majorly early on, it's very important.

Jed Baker: Three, four weeks, and I can't, shortness of my breath is my biggest symptom.

JH: That was key. I can't stress enough the significance of that, not only for the prevention of pneumonia or fluid buildup, but also for the development of your lungs, because they do collapse your lungs depending on your situation and how you went into the surgery. Were you on a rested heart, Jed?

Jed Baker: Yeah, they stopped my heart. I was on the bypass machine.

JH: Okay, so it's really critical that you're working with a spirometer. As difficult as it is and as much a pain in the butt it is, it's significant.

Jed Baker: I'll tell you, so is the walking and really breathing. Heavy walking is really equally good to clear whatever sort of mucus might be there and things like that. Yep, totally agree. I will tell you this, as I've been doing better and my exercise tolerance keeps going up. I had one glitch about two weeks into it.

I just woke up one morning and I had tachycardia. My heart was racing. It wasn't an arrhythmia, it was just stuck at around 125, 130, just sitting doing nothing. I went to the ER and at the instruction of the surgeon got checked out, heart rate came down, they discharged me, didn't get admitted and since then it hasn't happened. I was on a written medication for the first month of surgery, because your heart is irritable and angry and it does weird things in that first month of surgery. That was the only weird sort of heart rhythm. It wasn't a rhythm issue, it was just a high rate. I haven't had that since. But I will tell you, last week I did my first webinar again other than what I'm doing with you today. It was a three-hour talk.

JH: Oh, wow, that's a long conversation.

Jed Baker: It's a long time and I started playing music again too and doing all that. The talking is the hardest thing for me and somewhere in there I got out of breath and kept thinking in my head do I need to cancel this now? I couldn't have even attempted that pre-surgery. I couldn't have even done like 10 minutes of the talk. It was really getting hard, but it was three hours and it went away.

JH: I would say also over time, not overnight. You're nine weeks, nine weeks in a lifetime of healing. It's pretty remarkable.

Jed Baker: My surgeon said something really important to me, Dr. Burns, which rang in my ear. When I would tell him I still have a little shortness of breath, especially after eating, but it's not as bad, it goes away. He said, I don't think you're going to wake up one morning and you're just better, and I know that's the experience of some people on the Facebook site. He said it's going to be slow and gradual, and he's been right. Every day and every week I get better. I'm doing cardiac rehab, I'm exercising, I feel really strong, I'm playing the drums again, exercising a lot. I'm feeling pretty good right now, Jeff, honestly.

JH: I'm going to ask you to change hats for a second from the physical part of all of this, because you are a clinical psychologist, you have a little bit more familiarity with people, anxiety, trauma, which this certainly is. How did you address that mental part of it? How did you work yourself through it, knowing what you know?

Jed Baker: Let me start by saying, "Not well." My wife can tell you what a pain I must have been. More so than the baseline pain that I usually am to her, yeah, but the normal Jed.

JH: Now it's the Jed with an issue.

Jed Baker: I was certainly obsessing about every decision and every possible cause and I couldn't talk about anything else in some ways that easily. I also remember saying I went to see a concert and I was in the balcony, I had to walk up these steps. I couldn't catch my breath. I remember there was a psychologist friend of mine sitting by me and I said I don't want to live if this is the way. I don't want to live. He's someone who had some chronic illness too. He said something that rang true to me, which is, that's an important thing to say, to say out loud as a statement. Because this is an incredibly challenging period when I can't breathe and couldn't do anything without feeling like I'm going to choke and not be able to breathe here. Right? Someone validating that you know it's okay to feel like that, it's not okay to get stuck there. You have to have hope and it's something I preach in the work that I do, and I preach that because of a couple things. First of all, there's all this research with the kids that I work with autism.

One of my colleagues, Mark Duran, had done this sort of research, see what predicts aggressive behavior with kids with autism, and the best predictor was parental hope, parental optimism and that when parents have hope that prevents that aggressive behavior. Over time they get better outcomes when they're hopeful, and it wasn't how aggressive the kid was when they were three that predicted how aggressive they'd be at six. A wild kid isn't going to have to continue to be a wild kid. Parental optimism was the single best predictor, which is that parents were relentless in trying to find help for their kids. I know that. I also know the classic learned helplessness, which is what we all experience when we're having this bridge, and nobody knows how to help us and cardiologists are saying it's fine, you're just anxious and you get this sort of learned helplessness. The classic learned helpless experiment is you put a rat in a jar in water and they tread water for like, I don't know, maybe an hour, and then they sink. But if somebody comes to rescue the rat within the first hour and you put them back in the glass, which is just awful, they tread water for two days. Two days. We're treading water when we're stuck with something that nobody understands and we don't know how to fix it. We need people like you and we need the myocardial support group to take us out of the glass of water for a second. Give us a little more hope.

JH: Right.

Jed Baker: That gave me enough hope to figure out. There's got to be a solution to this, and I'm so much better as a result, and that's certainly what I would say to anybody going through this.

JH: Jed, it's not me, I'm just the conduit, it's you, it's all of you, it's everybody that participates in the program that gives us the opportunity to share for the benefit of the others who are where we were and we know what that's like. We know that sensation. We know that feeling. We know that mental state and I think the more we can share, the more we can tell, because every story is so unique, every situation is so unique, every bridge is so unique. No two are the same and the more stories people hear, the more one is going to be closer to that particular individual's story, to where they can say that's me. That's my symptom. I've got this. He's really helping me by sharing that, because now I know I'm not the unicorn sitting here in this group. Obviously, it's us. When it becomes us, it's our world, that's all there is, is us. You get very myopic in terms of the situation and to hear even somebody who's just close to what your situation is, it's like thank God. Okay, that's similar. I'm not alone.

Jed Baker: Let me say this too, because part of the agony of making the decision is on that support group. You get people who've been really successfully unroofed and are feeling great, but you're also more likely to get the people who are still having trouble. Yes, because those of us who get better, you stop looking at the Facebook group after a while perhaps, and that's hard to hear too.

I want to say something about that, because some of the people I've grown to sort of commiserate with and love and feel a brotherhood and a sisterhood with, they sometimes have complications after the unroofing. It happens, and sometimes they don't totally go away. They need to have hope too. Right? That's the thing that I practice in my clinical practice. You have to be a salesperson of hope, and my refrain is all problems can be solved or greatly improved if you can wait. That's the hardest part. Talk to the right person. You knock on every door. There are people who have pericarditis and it returns frequently for some people. Fortunately, I have not had any of that, but I know there's a solution for that too, and there are new medications coming out. You have to knock on every door. My cardiologist' office literally said to me, "We don't know much about myocardial bridges. You should continue to research that on the Internet and find the people that do."

I felt like I was Elaine on the Seinfeld show, where I was blacklisted from the cardiology office. Okay, here comes the anxious guy. Whatever he says, he's just anxious. It's not real.

JH: That happened to Lewis Merlin. The hospital said no more, you're done. You keep coming in here with these issues. You have nothing wrong with you.

Obviously, you have a stressful position. You're a psychologist, but you have an outlet as well.

Jed Baker: Yes. Music is a is a place where I can lose myself. I'm a drummer. Originally a jazz drummer but I also got to be in this soul sort of funk rock band. Tower of Power stuff, James Brown, things like that and we got to play in great dive bars. Unfortunately, when all this went on and they had lots of gigs to do, I kind of lost that position. I'm probably in the rotation again when they need a drummer. We're all of a certain age, so they get rotator cuff issues and whatever else. But I'm back to doing the jazz and I got to play just before I saw you today.

JH: I'm wondering if your surgeon's cool with this? He says okay, sternotomy, he's still in sternal precaution, yet you're moving around on the drums. You're all over the place!

Jed Baker: Well, I'll tell you at the sixth week mark, that was the last time I saw my surgeon unless I want to reach him again. I didn't really ask him. I will tell you this. I'm not lifting anything heavy here. These are drumsticks. They're light. I am moving and for the most part I'm trying to move but I'm not totally twisting, which I can still feel. I still have some rib soreness in one area.

JH: You're only nine weeks out. Jed it's a 12-week procedure, a 12-week process to heal. You've still got another three or four weeks!

Jed Baker: I'm not feeling any pain when I play or even after I play. I was never going to make a living doing that, but I'm happy to still get a chance that people will let me play with them.

JH: As we wrap up, one of the things I'm asking everybody who has gone through the procedure, for those who are in the process of making the decision, who have been diagnosed, and they're stuck. Sometimes it's stuck because they can't make a decision on whether they are going to go through a robotic process or a sternotomy. They're stuck because of the fear of the procedure, or they're just generally stuck because they can't get past the next steps. Maybe it's insurance, maybe it's travel, maybe it's family. What would you say to those people?

Jed Baker: First of all, there's got to be some people who do okay with medication for a long time because, given the number of people who have bridges, who, A, are not even symptomatic. Those of us who are symptomatic, I've seen some people on the site who try that, but when it gets to a point, as it has for many of us and for me, where I was not living my life anymore, then you have to elect to have this surgery. They're not demanding it; you're not going to die unless we do this tomorrow. That's different for some people, like yourself. If you're having a heart attack, you've got to do something, but it's a hard decision to make. It's agonizing. And who you're going to see, right?

Dr Schnittger said something that was very useful to me. I might not be able to pay to go to Stanford. She said look for a surgeon who's done tons of bypass surgeries, because then they are working with those small arteries all the time. Look for someone who's done at least five unroofings, where that's exclusively an unroofing and look for a surgeon who is on board with completely unroofing you, not partially. That made the decision a little bit easier about who to see and maybe could free up some of your listeners who are in places where maybe, like me, they couldn't get to Stanford, or they were turned down from Stanford. There are other surgeons who meet that criteria.

The other thing I want to say to people is the sternotomy. It didn't really hurt because there's not a lot of nerves in your bones, the nerves are in the muscles. There's some soreness around it, but I've got to say, other than the tubes being in me for that first day, it was not that painful. And although it's a long recovery, I would liken it to anybody who has to do some sort of major knee construction, reconstruction. It takes that kind of time. It's not as scary as it sounds.

I'll just say what I say to all of my clients and say to myself and live by. All problems can be solved, or at least greatly improved, if you can wait and talk to the right person.

EMILY TEDORE: A Ho Ho Holiday Like No Other

(The story of a mother's efforts to make it home for the holiday post-unroofing.)

Our story begins in the gym with a mother of two from the Sierra Nevada. Fresh from a period of maternal hiatus she was keen to regain her pre-pregnancy fitness. But that wasn't to be the case as she was struck by an unfamiliar, chest-clenching sensation. Unlike anything she'd felt before, it sent her into high alert.

Remembering a friend who had suffered a heart attack, she quickly dialed 911. Upon arrival, the paramedics administered an EKG and noted something was off. As her chest pain persisted, she found herself navigating medical uncertainty. A seemingly endless night of anxiety ensued as medical professionals performed a series of tests, from blood work to CT scans, only to conclude that "everything looks fine." As she grappled with her escalating pain, she felt her concerns being met with skepticism. Her story, as every other, takes some very unique twists and turns not unlike a windy mountain road in the region where she resides.

Jeff Holden (Host): Emily Tedore is a 39-year-old mother of two daughters, four and 15. She lives with her partner in the beautiful Sierra Nevada, at the base of Lake Tahoe and folks, this is a spectacularly beautiful setting, I promise you. She's originally from Iowa but moved out to the west in the mid-90s, loves most anything outdoors, including mountain biking, hiking, fishing and snow skiing. She tells me she bakes a mean sourdough loaf and has just started to learn how to do canning. I hope I'll get to experience that at some point. She loves the winter and snow, the two things that made me leave the Midwest, and is looking forward to getting back to snow skiing and teaching her four-year-old for the first time, which would not have been possible if she hadn't been recently unroofed. She works full-time and is also currently working toward her master's degree in communications.

Emily, what was it that began your journey toward an unroofing procedure? What started this whole process for you?

Emily Tedore (Guest): I had just recently started back going to the gym and exercising after having had my daughter. Of course, as moms, we want to get back in shape after not exercising for a while. I was at the gym, and I was doing some weighted lunges, a normal exercise, nothing crazy. As soon as I had set down the weights, my entire chest got extremely tight. This is something I had never experienced before. I thought maybe I pulled a muscle. I started stretching and feeling and I was like, nah, this is something more than just a muscle, like something's not right. I had had a friend, a woman, who had had another heart issue. She had had a heart attack. I thought of her instantly and I thought maybe I had damaged my heart or something had happened. I got very concerned and walked out of the gym and I called 911. The ambulance came. They did an EKG and said well, my EKG looks a little off. They didn't really tell me what it was. We should probably just take you to the ER to run some more tests to make sure nothing more serious is happening. Off I went to the ER in the ambulance and while I was in the ambulance, they had given me, I believe it's nitro. It's the one you put under your tongue. They said if this helps, then it probably is something to do with your heart. It helped. I got very concerned because prior to that I had not had any heart issues. I was a relatively healthy person.

Once we got there, they did blood work and they said oh, your blood work looks fine, everything's fine, the normal ER response. Are you sure you didn't pull a muscle? Are you sure you're not having anxiety? I said no, no, I'm still having this really bad pain. They did an echocardiogram and a CT scan and said everything looks fine. I'm telling them it's not getting better; it's not getting better. They finally gave me morphine and, I think, Valium. Slowly it started to subside and my chest wasn't as tight. It was funny because right after the pain had kind of subsided, I started having all these heart palpitations. I knew what those were. They're pretty common in most adults. I'm having a bunch of them right now and they go oh well, that's normal for adults, that's a normal thing to have. They're happening back-to-back-to-back. Finally, they just said we don't know what's wrong with you, everything's fine. It's probably 2 AM, they did one last blood work, and I came back with elevated troponin levels, which was indicative of a heart attack. They said it was a moderate level, so not mild, but not severe. Then it got more serious. They put me on the blood thinners and then they decided that they were going to do the heart cath the next morning. That was a really long, anxiety-filled night. The next day they took me into the cath lab. They did the cath through my wrist and they said we see a myocardial bridge in there, but those are benign, nothing to worry about. We do see that one wall of your ventricle was ballooning a little bit. We believe this is Takotsubo (also called "broken heart" syndrome, a temporary weakening of the heart muscle). This is something that I guess is common in women. By that time, I felt better. I felt great. My heart function was actually a little above average. My heart function is still really good and strong. They said, oh, Takotsubo and they sent me on my way. They gave me metoprolol and aspirin and said follow up with your cardiologist. That's where I ended up.

JH: I'm concerned with the troponin level.

Emily Tedore: They just said oh yeah, you had a heart attack, and this is kind of what we think actually what it was. It really wasn't much of an answer. It wasn't super reassuring at all for me.

JH: That got you through the first incident with a hospital visit, right? Roughly two days in, how long ago was this?

Emily Tedore: This was in September of 2021.

JH: Then they identified the bridge, which is a step in the right direction. What happened then? What was the next step? It could have been oh, everything's fine, happy life, I'm all good. Nothing happened to cause you to continue to go down a path of looking for something to address. What happened next?

Emily Tedore: Then I had my follow-up appointment with my cardiologist and well, it actually ended up being a nurse practitioner that was there. It wasn't the cardiologist. She said because I was just expressing to her how worried I was and how I was having anxiety about it, feeling stressed, couldn't exercise, couldn't do anything, she said, I'm going to refer you over to a different cardiologist within our group. It's a group of cardiologists. She's around your age; she's a nice woman. She works up at the university and they do a lot of different studies and I think you would be a better fit with her than the gentleman that I had seen in the ER. I scheduled that appointment and then when that appointment came along, I had moved on from it. I had accepted it. I didn't have any other symptoms. I felt back to my normal self. I went into that appointment, and she came on pretty strong and she said I don't believe that you had Takotsubo. She said your troponin levels are much higher than a Takotsubo event. Your heart function was still well and strong and normally with a Takotsubo, the heart function will go down. She said "I really want to look at that bridge and I want to make sure that that bridge in your heart was not what caused this. That this isn't something that could happen again in the future. You are a mom. You're still young. I don't want you to have problems. I want to send you for a series of tests." She made appointments for another CT scan and an MRI of my heart. Long story short, everything came back looking good on all those tests, except the MRI did show scar tissue and damage on my heart from that one event. That was very alarming to me. Of course, I started going down a Google hole, which I never recommend. You get scar tissue on your heart, and your heart doesn't really heal itself, according to my Google search. I was very concerned and she says well, I wouldn't worry too much about it. Your heart function is still really well, you feel good and that's all good.

They kept me on the heart medication and she added one additional medication that she thought may help with lowering my blood pressure. I think my blood pressure was high because of the anxiety surrounding everything that was going on. I was having a lot of anxiety. She put me on another medication. I stayed on the metoprolol. I stayed on baby aspirin, and she also has me on a statin just for preventative measures. After all the results came back, she said, I want to go ahead and refer you to Stanford. This is around the time that I had found the myocardial bridge Facebook group. I had started looking on there and I had heard Stanford mentioned a few times but I hadn't gone down researching it significantly on the group yet until she said I want to refer you. She sent in my referral and I didn't hear back for probably a month or so.

JH: The novelty of having an episode and then going to a cardiologist who actually recognizes the bridge as something symptomatic in the first step is amazing. You may be one of a few people on our Facebook group that was connected, post-incident, to your first episode. Three steps were symptom, major symptom, as you find out after the fact, because it caused a little bit of damage, and then to a cardiologist who recognizes a bridge is symptomatic, directly to the next step of Stanford. In so many cases it takes three, four, five different steps and months, in some cases, years, for people.

Emily Tedore: Yes, I was very lucky and I will happily share her name. Her name is Dr. Laurel Toft out of Carson Tahoe cardiology. She is also a professor at the medical school at the University of Nevada, Reno. She only sees patients one day a week at Carson Tahoe and then she is actually a teacher up at UNR, which is why I believe she probably knew so much about Stanford. We are fairly close to Stanford. I was very lucky.

JH: She's a great doctor. So the next thing you know, you're in the process of referral to Stanford. What happens from there?

Emily Tedore: That was a big waiting game. I waited about a month or so and then a woman named Joy at Stanford reached out to me and she requested all my medical records, which then I got together. I sent them down to Stanford. It was about another week or two. They got back to me and said that you would be a candidate to come down and have further testing done. Of course, they don't tell you if you'll have surgery or not, because everyone is so different. That was probably in April or May. She didn't have a date for me until it was mid-summer. She finally gave me a date in December. It was a pretty good chunk of time until I was actually on their calendar. They're so busy, but once I was on their calendar, they're super responsive, super helpful. Stanford is most amazing. I haven't been to a lot of hospitals, but they interact with you, they talk to you, answer any questions, you have their app, everything is great. They got me on their calendar and unfortunately for me, it was December 12th when I would go down there. I looked at the calendar and I was like holy cow; I'm potentially having heart surgery right before Christmas. As a mom, any moms know, that's not a good time for anything to be scheduled. That was stressful. But our health comes first.

JH: You have two children in the Santa space at this time too, so you definitely don't want to be missing it. We're very similar in terms of timing. Mine was January 4th. My diagnosis and provocative test were done the day after Thanksgiving. I spent Thanksgiving at Stanford in the hospital so I was prepped and ready to go on Friday. After the testing they said, okay, yes, we're going to schedule you. I said, okay, when? Next week? I'm ready. Right? It would have been in that year. It would have been the year in 2021 had we been able to get everybody coordinated, but one of the doctors was going on vacation and I had a couple of different complications that need to be taken care of. It ended up being January 4th, but I was just saying bring it on. My kids are grown and gone. Sooner is better than later. Yours was roughly, what was that, September to December, almost a year later?

Emily Tedore: Yes.

JH: Over a year you had this, this anxiety. You were on some medication, not really knowing what's going to happen, but you didn't have any other significant episodes over the course of that time.

Emily Tedore: No, I didn't. I was very nervous about exercising or pushing myself, and so my doctor said go ahead and keep your heart rate below 140. That way you feel comfortable. Which was hard. Being someone who was active and having an active family around me, to try and monitor my heart rate and keep it low was really tricky, but ultimately, I think it was good because it helped relieve anxiety. This happened while I was exercising. I was very nervous to go out and push myself. Anyone who mountain bikes or road bikes knows your heart rate can get pretty wild. You know it can. It can spike up there pretty high, biking. I'm not going to do any of that. I'm going to hold off. I'm going to sit tight until I can get down to Stanford. I ended up having surgery December 22nd and was released from the hospital on the 26th. It was the day after Christmas Day.

JH: Oh my gosh, so you did do it.

Emily Tedore: Yes.

JH: What a Christmas present.

Emily Tedore: Yeah. Luckily, I have a really good family. My kids ended up staying here in Nevada with Marco, my partner, their dad. He has a huge family. Everyone chipped in and took care of the girls and, of course, FaceTime. I FaceTime them all the time. My mom went down to Stanford with me and we stayed in Sunnyvale. We tried to enjoy ourselves, did

Christmas shopping and everything else. I brought the Christmas gifts down to Stanford because we thought maybe they would be able to come down after I had the surgery and was released into Christmas down there. Unfortunately, they all got sick and so I said stay home. I don't want you here. Santa came on New Year's Eve when I got back home, so it was fine.

JH: Let me ask you, you have your heart attack. You go through the process of anxiety, wait, wait, wait, wait. You finally get in for your provocative testing and they do identify it, obviously something significant enough to say, even though she's not severely symptomatic, we need to address this and take care of it. Do you know any of the details, the general details of what your bridge was like? Why they thought that it needed to be addressed so quickly?

Emily Tedore: I think their concern was that while you're not really symptomatic, it was how do you feel? I feel okay, but I haven't been pushing myself. The bridge itself was not that long, but it was so deep that it did go down into the ventricle. It was a real tight, tight little bridge there. When they did go in and they did the cath where they go and they increase, I don't know the technical terms, forgive me, but they increase your heart rate, when they do that, I got the same extreme pain, spasms in my chest. When they did that, I you know you're sedated, but I was going, oh, it hurt. It was the same sensation as before. Dr. Schnittger said yes, you have severe endothelial dysfunction. You would definitely be a candidate for surgery. Although it was hard, because Dr. Boyd put the ball in my court. He said you don't suffer with symptoms every day, but you do have the endothelial dysfunction. I don't know how to make that decision. How do you decide?

My mom asked if I can live with the amount of anxiety I've been having for the last year and fear of exercising and fear of this happening again? Can you keep living that way? I said no and we said okay, let's do it, let's do the surgery. I knew I couldn't keep living so scared of everything all the time, and the anxiety and everything that goes along with this heart issue, the rest of my life worried all the time. I'm so active and I don't want to be held back.

JH: One of the things that a lot of the doctors will tell you is that stress causes even more complications, especially if you have a bridge, and no bridge gets better over time.

Emily Tedore: Right, yes.

JH: The fact that you were able to get it done at this young age, before you became either debilitated by symptoms or caused even more damage to the heart, I think that was a wise decision.

Emily Tedore: Yes, and like you said, it doesn't go away, it doesn't get better, it can only potentially get worse over time. We went for it when we were down there. We don't want to have to do this again if I continue to have problems or I develop more problems. We just want to get it taken care of and get it done and get back to living life. My blood pressure had crept up so much just from the stress of everything. Am I having surgery? Am I not having surgery? What's going to happen? When am I having it? Am I going to have another heart attack? I just wanted to get better and get past it.

JH: It's so true about that heart attack concern. I think we all experience it. If something happens, I had a heart attack, you had a heart attack. Many of the people had some sort of a myocardial infarction on the Facebook group. Knowing they have a bridge, the question becomes, is the next one going to be devastating? Am I going to get severe damage? Am I going to die? You just don't know. That uncertainty, if you didn't have anxiety before, the uncertainty of it, will create the anxiety that is again a stressor which causes problems in the long run. Over the grand scheme of things, yes, we should take care of it. You have a choice. Your symptoms aren't that bad. You're not getting it every day, but you know, in two, three, four years then it becomes every day. Right now, you're back to where you started and now you may have some further damage because you waited.

Emily Tedore: Exactly, exactly.

JH: So, post-surgery, tell us what that was like. You get home, it's a new year, happy new year!

Emily Tedore: Actually, right after you have surgery, you're in the hospital and of course I think a lot of people have the low blood pressure issue right out of surgery. We dealt with that. Then you get breathless and tired. Once they figure out your pain levels, I think they put me on oxycodone and that helped, but it made me feel so groggy. As soon as I could stop taking that, I did because I hated the drunken, yucky feel of it. I couldn't text on my phone because I couldn't *see* my phone. It wasn't very much fun but it helped with the pain.

If you know you have the option to get the epidural in your back, I definitely recommend that because it really helps pain-wise, to be able to take your deep breaths to get oxygen into your lungs. If you go to Stanford, they tell you all that. I felt like even when I wasn't using my little machine that they give you to breathe, I was always trying to take really deep breaths and always trying to cough out any junk that was in there. I would breathe in until the point it was painful, and then I would let my breath out. I would do it all the time, even when I wasn't using the machine. I felt like that helped a lot with not getting a lot of fluid buildup. I was always doing that in the hospital getting up, walking, you're still very breathless, even when you release from the hospital. It was hard to even hold a conversation for very long because I couldn't catch my breath. I'm talking on the phone and it wasn't great. But every single day it would get better and better. It was like every day you'd feel a little bit better, every day a little bit better. We did our walking exercises that Stanford gives you that they're very specific on. Okay, every day you need to go out and walk and, being someone who uses the Strava app for tracking physical exercise, I was capturing my walk around the hotel room because I was just trying to get myself feeling better and getting in a mindset of getting better.

When we get back home, there was a horrible storm that hit on New Year's Eve in Nevada and we almost did not make it back over the pass driving home. They were slowly shutting it down. There are three different highways to get over the mountain and we saw them shut down. We're already on our way and we checked out of the hotel, my mom's driving my car home and finally it's the last highway. We see that it gets shut down, the one we're on, and they're shutting it down for avalanche control. My mom says we're going for it. We're not letting this stop us, we're getting home. At that point, we had been down there for three and a half weeks and we were just ready to be home. It was probably not the smartest, but we just went for it. We let them clear avalanches and we made it home in a pretty hairy snowstorm.

Once I was home, I wasn't sure how I would be able to help with my little one, because at that point she was three. I still had family help that would come over and help do the harder things like bath time and those things. I can't lift her. Luckily, she was really good, she was very sweet and very patient with me. I had lots of family help.

I could do a lot of things. I could wash dishes, I could sort of make dinner, as long as I was doing the sternal precautions where you keep your elbows in. You're in the tube. I wasn't reaching out and lifting heavy things. I could do mostly anything. There were, of course, times where I would get that zing through my sternum and I'm like, okay, listen to my body, back off. I didn't want to just sit there like a lump on a log and do nothing. I wanted to stay moving, keep. I wanted to get better.

JH: What you just said is really, really important for anybody that's in the process of, or about to have the surgery with a sternotomy. That is, post-surgery, be active. And I'm not talking about go out and try to run or something, just be active. Do something. Get up. Don't sit on the couch and take Oxy because it hurts, right? Work your body to an improvement every day, over whatever number of steps it is. If you do 50, do 100. If you do 100, do 150, but do something and continue to do something.

I do want to go back for a second on the spirometer, that little breathing device, which is a pain. We all hate it. They say you've got to use it. It's so significant because it's there for two things: the prevention of pneumonia and also to get your lung expansion back, because during a sternotomy they collapse the lungs and it's really important that you do that so that when you come back, you're back to where you were, as opposed to with a diminished lung capacity or, worse yet, some sort of bronchial issue or pneumonia. That's the last thing you want when you have a sternotomy.

You sound like you're doing pretty good. You're into January now and you're functioning, starting to work your way outside the tube as the months go along. Did you notice anything different? You were so super cautious pre-surgery and now, all of a sudden, you're doing it, and you go wow, I wouldn't even have done that before because I was so concerned. Here I am doing it and it's second nature, like it used to be?

Emily Tedore: Yes. Really, any movement and exercise that I had started to incorporate. We had gotten a huge blizzard. We had snow on the ground for weeks and weeks and I would go out and I'd put my Apple Watch on, put a podcast in my ear, and walk in my snow boots in the snow. That way I was getting my walking in, and it was nice to not constantly be staring at my heart rate on my Apple Watch going, "Where is it?" That was one thing they taught me. After when they released me from the hospital, I had a higher heart rate. My heart rate, my resting heart rate was probably like in the 90s to 100s and one of the doctors said maybe that's just your new resting heart rate. No, that's kind of high. That's weird. He was like, I don't know, don't stare at your Apple Watch. Don't obsess over it, just go back to going about your day, don't look at it and see what happens. I did that and, sure enough, it just started to go down. It's like the staring at it just makes your heart rate go up and then you start fixating on it and so I started walking. My heart rate came down. I started just being more active. I didn't really do anything outside of walking until I had gone to the cardiac rehab where they pushed me harder. I was waiting to do anything harder than walking until I got monitored and did that program.

JH: Tell me a little bit about the emotional part of it for you. We're always concerned about what the reality of this is going to be and we don't know, no matter how many people tell you, nobody's ever died on the table. It's a pretty safe surgery. We know what we're doing. Yeah, that's good. You're cutting my chest open to mess with my heart. So you go into the surgery and you come out of it. Where's your head on that? What were you thinking? What was going through your mind? Family, all that. How are you dealing with it? I know a lot of people ask the question as they get concerned or fearful about the surgery to the point that we're almost paralyzed.

Emily Tedore: Right. I would definitely say I was in the high anxiety, fear, paralyzed state for a long time. Like I had said, my blood pressure crept up quite a bit from anxiety. My cardiologist, even she prescribed me an anti-anxiety medication, but I never ended up taking it because I was going to deal with this on my own. One of the blood pressure medications that they had given me, though, did help with the anxiety, so I hung in there with that.

Really, I think a big part of this, too, is the emotional stress it takes on people. It's hard, even outside of the symptoms you have. Mentally it's a very stressful thing, and it doesn't help that there isn't a lot of knowledge about it. I think the Facebook group is amazing. I do want to mention a gal that I met on there. Her name is Casey. She was my saving grace to this whole process. I don't know her outside of the Facebook group that we have, but she started messaging me and we talked almost every single day leading up into my trip to Stanford. When I was down at Stanford, we talked every single day. She is a mom. She has a little toddler, and she was just a huge support system. It's hard to talk to family and friends because they don't understand the issue with the heart a lot of times. They don't understand what you're going through, they don't understand a lot of it. It's hard to vent to family and friends. If you can find someone within the community of people who have this issue, someone within the Facebook group that you can talk to, you can message me if you're on the Facebook group and I can I feel like that helped a lot.

There was another gentleman, I don't remember his name. I spoke to him leading up to surgery. He had surgery at Stanford and then after the fact, I had spoken to a few other people who went through surgery after me. I was a support to them and so having that community of people who've been through it, really helped with my anxiety.

Casey helped tremendously with me. It was every day I was at Stanford. We were talking and she was saying you're fine, you're going to be fine, it's not a big deal and that's what I needed to hear. I get wound up in my mind easily and she would just talk me down. You'll be fine, you'll be back home and doing what you want in no time. That helped with me a lot. Post, once I had the surgery, it was like that weight was completely lifted off my shoulders. I made it through surgery. Once you get through the waking up with the breathing tube, which I feel like they should warn you about ahead of time since that was kind of stressful, but you get through it and you look back on it and go, ok, that sucked but keep moving forward. Stay positive. Once I had surgery, like I said, I just felt so much better.

JH: All those tubes suck, yes, the breathing tube, the chest tubes yes, those three, yes.

Emily Tedore: Once they take the chest tubes out, you're like a whole new person. It was like all right, let's go.

JH: If there's one thing in your perspective, now that you're unroofed and you've been able to exercise, you've got your former self back in terms of capability, and things that you're doing, what would you say it is? Is there something that you can say, this is really different because I've been through this and it's probably the most significant part of it? Not just the fact that we went through it and had our chest ripped open and all that, but the emotional part of it, the thing you look at from life a little bit differently, if you do. Is there something that you're left with now that you've had this opportunity? Let's call it a rebirth, because you don't have to worry about that heart situation.

Emily Tedore: Yes. I think with any huge medical issue you always think in your head, well, I'm healthy, nothing's going to happen to me. Then, when something happens to you, you can get a scary diagnosis. It really changes your perspective on life. Without good health, it's very scary. You can't really do much without having your health on track. I have so much more appreciation for all the parts of me that work well and I'm so thankful. I'm really focused on eating well and exercising and taking good care of myself now. Before, it's like, oh, I'm healthy, I'm fine. You never know when something's going to happen big or you're going to have a heart attack. Nobody's immune to something like a big life health event happening. Now I really appreciate all the moments. It's cliche to say, but you enjoy every moment of life because you just don't know when something's going to happen. I enjoy every moment with my kids and every moment outside. I enjoy doing the things I love, because when you can't do those for a year, it really puts perspective on everything. People who complain about exercising, I think to myself, oh, you don't know what it's like to not be able to exercise. That's huge, like someone telling you OK, you can't exercise when people complain about exercising, you have a whole new appreciation of being able to get your heart rate up there and sweat and feel good and do all those things. That's been huge for me.

JH: Please, please, let me go out and torture myself. I would love to. Yes, don't tell me I can't. I want to do that.

Emily Tedore: Yes, maybe not the level that you did, Jeff, but I don't know.

JH: I'll share that with people, and not so much the Death Ride, but that's kind of what connected us. I was going for a ride in the Sierra and Emily, you had seen it, and you said, I live there. I volunteer for that ride for the riders coming through. I think it's with your daughter's riding club, right?

Emily Tedore: Yes, my daughter's on a mountain bike team. You say it's a little ride, but the Death Ride is insane. You know how many feet of climbing. I mean, if you've ever ridden a bike and you know the elevation game on a bike, it's huge what you did. I'm amazed that you did it. But, yes, my daughter volunteers for your ride. We help and do the bike corral, and they help with the nutrition stations of the ride. That's how we connected.

JH: Unfortunately, this was the one year I'm doing the ride and you're on vacation.

Emily Tedore: Right, we ended up going out of town. Next year.

JH: I will tell you I could have used the motivation at about the turn where we start to head back.

Emily Tedore: Yeah, I bet.

JH: You've got an anniversary coming up, which I think is really cool. We call it a second birthday, whatever you want. It happens to be right around Christmas on top of it, and it's so cool to think that last year you were in the hospital.

Emily Tedore: Right.

JH: You didn't get to celebrate Christmas with the family at home. This year it's a whole different deal. You're going to be home. You're going to be well and I just I feel so good about it that you're going to get to experience it without having the anxiety and the worry of what might be wrong with me. Happy anniversary, Merry Christmas and all that. The other part of it that's really neat is now you have the ability to go out and play with your kids again and do the things that you love to do, to teach them that mom can be with them to do it.

Emily Tedore: Exactly yes, we're very excited to get back out skiing.

JH: And now we just have to hope for some snow.

Emily Tedore: Yes.

RAISUL ISLAM: A Father's Travel From Bangladesh To California

(An unusual benefit of being a student at Stanford when you have access to good care.)

You can only imagine my excitement at seeing a Stanford University email address show up in my inbox for a guest on my podcast, Imperfect Heart. Especially from a gentleman with "Dr." preceding his name. Could I really have a Stanford doctor reaching out to be on the program? A Stanford doctor with a myocardial bridge? I can't wait. This will be great!

Well, that wasn't quite the case, but the story is every bit as good as I might have expected. This was a Stanford doctor, but his doctorate is in electrical engineering. And while he got his degree from Stanford, he's from Bangladesh. Yes, let your imagination run. How is it that a gentleman with a great story to share just happens to travel across the world and end up at the very university that not only provides his degree but is also the same place that can correct his, unbeknownst at the time, life threatening condition? We'll let him share it with us.

Having grown up in Dhaka, the capital of Bangladesh, Raisul Islam studied electrical and electronic engineering at Bangladesh University. In 2011, he moved to Stanford University to pursue his doctorate with a focus on ultra-thin solar cell technology, graduated in 2017 and currently works for a startup company that aims to revolutionize high-speed, highly scalable memory technology.

Jeff Holden (Host): So many of our listeners have unique, diverse, and compelling stories. Yours is certainly that. You are no stranger to an awareness that something may not have been right with you for quite some time. I'm talking about starting all the way back in Bangladesh. Can you tell us a little bit about that?

Raisul Islam (Guest): Yes, I think it all started when I was in high school, maybe in 11th grade or 12th grade. There was one day when I just had palpitations and without any stressor or anything. It just started on its own. I wasn't sure what had gone wrong, because I was having this pounding sensation in my chest. My blood pressure was significantly higher. My heart rate was 160 without even doing anything, no exercise or anything. That was the beginning of what I would call the awareness of these symptoms. After that I was seen by doctors, many doctors. And since I was very young then, nobody actually looked into the heart initially. They thought, okay, this is probably some kidney issue. I got all sorts of tests regarding my kidneys and the kidney function was normal. I still have that high blood pressure and the doctors prescribing this and that medication to control it and it responded well most of the time. Then the doctors say that you don't have to continue these medications for long. Probably, it's anxiety. I was even referred to see a psychiatrist as well. It's always been said, okay, it's just anxiety. You are probably having anxiety; you are probably going through transitions in your life. That's what causing it. There is nothing wrong with you.

JH: We hear that so, so often from so many people that it's anxiety or it's stress, right? Or it's some other disorder.

Raisul Islam: The thing is, I was told anxiety so many times regarding these episodes of palpitations that I, at some point, grew fed up with it. I thought like, okay, if it really is anxiety, then I'll probably not think about it ever again. In 2011, when I decided to come to the U.S. from Bangladesh, I did not bring any of my medical records with me. I thought, okay, I'm going to forget that this happened, and if I do that, maybe then I don't have to think about it again.

JH: It'll be a fresh start. You thought, you were going to get a fresh start, but it didn't quite work that way.

Raisul Islam: It did not work that way. Not at all. What happened is that after I came to Stanford, for many reasons, for typical flu, fever, cough, this and that, I went to see local doctors, the primary care physicians in the campus health center. Every time I go there, they had my vitals recorded. I had probably around towards, I think in the 2012, I had like five consecutive visits where my blood pressure came out to be high. Quite high actually, for my age. The doctor told me, hey, it seems like you are continuously having this high blood pressure problem, and I know that you probably don't have any history, so we might want to check you out. Then I actually told them, no, I actually did not tell you all my story. I actually had a little bit of history, but I thought I did not have it anymore. The issue is that my blood pressure has been high for so long, for so many years that 140 over 90, I don't even feel it in my body

JH: Oh boy.

Raisul Islam: Unless it goes like really high, above 150, diastolic 110, then I probably feel something, but I'm so used to it, that 140, 90, I don't even register it, so I don't complain about it, and that's why it has gotten silent. It remains silent for a while. Then the doctor said, you know, now that I can see it, I measure it. You should get a test again. She sent me back to Stanford Hospital and to the nephrology department. Basically, to a kidney doctor. She did all the testing for kidneys and it came back negative. She just prescribed me a water pill, diuretic for controlling my blood pressure. What happened was that it did not suit my body too well because it actually caused my potassium level to deplete too much, too fast.

There was a specific event that almost killed me because the potassium level was low, significantly. When it happened the night before, I actually ate a little bit of a salty snack, and in the morning I had the first episode or feeling of what it's like to have a heart attack. The severe chest pain. I could not even breathe. I had severe shortness of breath and I remember I was on campus that time and I called 911, EMTs came, and they hooked me up with a monitor. I was looking at their faces. It was not great. I could see they were not happy. They were worried about what they're seeing on the monitor. There was a little bit of an ST elevation within, which indicates that there could be an ischemia (reduced blood flow). But it was, at that time, luckily, I did not have a heart attack. It was because of the depletion of the potassium. They took me to the hospital; they did all the workup to rule out everything. Then again, I'm kind of on my own, but what happened was that after that, I got another referral to cardiology because the medication, the diuretic wasn't working. This is the first time I got like a little bit more focused towards the cardiac treatment plan that I first started getting. I was referred to Dr. John Schroeder of Stanford. He is a very prominent cardiologist and he's very, very experienced. At that time there was no thought or even any discussion of myocardial bridge. It's all like, okay, you have high blood pressure. Around that time he did all the blood work, it came out that my lipid profile is also too high. My LDL is high. My HDL is significantly low. In fact, I probably have never had a test where I get HDL high no matter how much good cholesterol I take. He said, you know, you probably have a bad gene, so you are at high risk because your cholesterol level is way off and you have high blood pressure. You have two risk factors, although you don't have any family history. I'm going to get you hooked up on a blood pressure medication and you have to take it properly and continuously along with a statin

JH: Lipitor.

Raisul Islam: Yeah. Initially I was on Atorvastatin a few months. I developed some side effects to it, muscle cramps, so I moved to Crestor. And then what he did, based on my experiences at ER, on the notes of the ER, he started me on Diltiazem, a calcium channel blocker. Luckily, calcium channel blocker is also a very popular treatment, or the first line or medication treatment for myocardial bridge as well.

JH: Yes. For Vasospasms,

Raisul Islam: Yes. To take care of the vasospasm.

JH: Yep. I know that one well. Same situation.

Raisul Islam: Right. A lot of the myocardial bridge patients also have endothelial dysfunction, which causes vasospasms and I have that too. Diltiazem actually helped quite a bit. My blood pressure was good. My heart rate was also, most of the time in the resting period, relatively low. So I stopped going back and forth to the ER towards the end of 2013. I thought, okay, this is fine. Initially I was seeing Dr. Schroeder often, then after a while, starting in 2014, I was seeing him like every six months and probably around 2017ish, I started seeing him once a year because everything was working fine. He had to increase the dose once because the blood pressure wasn't getting fully controlled, but it was more or less fine and I was able to do most of my stuff I was able to do. I was able to play soccer and everything. All the symptoms came back again pretty recently, actually, in the last few years.

JH: So, even though your blood pressure had been lowered and you were on the medication, everything was seemingly going well until it wasn't.

Raisul Islam: Before this cardiac history started coming back again around 2019, I was also diagnosed with an autoimmune disease. I was diagnosed with psoriatic arthritis. That's a different story and the longer story, but the gist of that was that I told Dr. Schroeder about it, about the diagnosis. He said, you now have another risk factor for a cardiac event, so we are going to increase your cholesterol medication. He added one more cholesterol medication. He said now your LDL cutoff should be even lower. You need to maintain a strict regimen of LDL. I started doing that. One of the things about the psoriatic arthritis is that besides joint pains it comes and goes. It has its flare and I was on the treatment. It was responding well. Occasionally after 2019, specifically around 2020, I started having these episodes of extreme tiredness, like extreme fatigue. And there is no explanation of why this fatigue would be there. I don't know if you have ever experienced this kind of fatigue, but if someone has not experienced it, it's really hard to explain to them.

JH: Yes.

Raisul Islam: I was very surprised at what is happening because my joint pains were gone and I was telling my rheumatologist that, hey, you know, maybe I have these, some of these, you know, tiredness, some of this flare-up is still coming. She said no, your joints seem to be fine. I'm not sure what is causing it. In 2020 I was going through another big change in my life. I was expecting my first baby. My first baby was born towards the end of 2020.

JH: Congratulations!

Raisul Islam: Thank you. And so, there have been a lot of transitions, a lot of things going on. After the baby was born, there were a lot of sleepless nights.

JH: Yes. And stressors and everything else.

Raisul Islam: Yes. It added lot of stress. I attributed everything to those stressors, to those sleepless nights and 2021, kept on building up, and kept building up, meaning the experience of fatigue.

JH: Okay. How was the chest? Any chest pain or unusual symptoms?

Raisul Islam: Now that I don't have chest pain, now that I don't have anything after the surgery, I feel so much better. I can feel that maybe I had heaviness in my chest. I always thought, okay, maybe I'm just too stressed. This is probably an anxiety attack or something because there is a heaviness to it. It's not a pain, but it's feels like I have something stuck on my chest. I could not get it off of my chest. Something heavy is on my chest. This is also very typical of anxiety, so I just thought like, okay, the fatigue, and then this heaviness is all about all about all the anxiety I'm going through until 2022.

The first time I actually collapsed, it was in July. I was in a grocery store and I just fell. I didn't know what happened. I was almost passed out but I could regain my consciousness very quickly. I did not have any control of over my body. That's the first time. It was in July of 2022. And I thought, okay, I was probably very tired or dehydrated, so I took electrolytes, water, fluids. Next day, the same thing happened again.

JH: Oh my.

Raisul Islam: Yeah. Yeah. Then I went to the ER for the first time with this, and at the same time I sent a message to Dr. Schroeder that, hey, I'm having this problem. It was the local ER. They ran all sorts of tests; EKG was always at the borderline. I think it was not very significant, at least at that time. All the cardiac enzymes were normal and then there were no rhythm issues that they could find. Imaging, mostly the x-rays, everything looked normal.

JH: It's interesting that you didn't have any arrhythmia, because that tends to be common with the condition.

Raisul Islam: No, I did not have any arrhythmia, luckily. Then I started seeing that my heart rate again, started shooting back up in the subsequent days since my ER visits. I saw Dr. Schroeder again after a long time, and he said, okay, maybe the diltiazem is not working. So let me give you a different calcium channel blocker, Amlodipine. It didn't work either. I still have this dizziness. By that time, I was kind of careful. It did not result in any falls, but it almost felt like the same. Then he stopped calcium channel altogether. Each and every week I was on a new medication. I started with amlodipine and then carvedilol, and then Metoprolol. Every drug I was trialing for one week or two weeks. I had a video call with him and it all seems like something is maybe 20% better, but I still have chest pain. Something is maybe 50% better, but I still have chest pain. Dr. Schroeder seems to be concerned. He said you should not have any chest pain. That's the point. You should not have any chest pains. If that is the case, then let's see what's going on. That's the first time, I think around August or end of July or early August he prescribed or referred me for a CT scan, CT and angiogram.

The report was mixed, had a lot of issues. It found plaque on the LAD, which is common for people with myocardial bridge. Then there was a myocardial bridge as well. The radiologist actually pointed out that there is a grade three myocardial bridge. The radiologist did not put any numbers there. I think grade-three is kind of deep, like fully immersed into the muscle. I read about it. Dr. Schroeder did not seem to be too concerned about the bridge. He was mostly concerned about the plaque because the plaque, it was mentioned in the report that the plaque was significant. 50% to 69%. It is significant for the age, but it is still not critical to have an intervention, right? For that, they require it to be above 70%. It is still not critical. I started on some aspirin as well, just to make sure that there is no blood clot. Then, in the middle of August, I had, again, these fully blown heart attack-like symptoms. I was taken to the Stanford Hospital at that time. I live 30 minutes from Stanford campus now, but my wife still drove me to Stanford Hospital because Dr. Schroeder told me you should always come to Stanford Hospital because that's where all your doctors are. I went there and they admitted me immediately because there was a CT scan that shows a 50% block. They thought this is definitely a heart attack. Luckily it was not a heart attack, but it still was a significant issue. Finally, since that hospital visit, I was referred to the myocardial bridge clinic because in that hospital stay, they did the full heart cath.

JH: So you had a provocative test?

Raisul Islam: Not a provocative, just an invasive angiogram. They checked whether the arteries were open or not, whether there is any obstructive coronary artery disease or not. These blocks, or these plaques were not blocking. It was clear. The doctors there, the attending physician told me, you don't have anything. You don't have an issue. You don't have to worry. Then I asked her what about the myocardial bridge? She said that it was hard to quote but that it was a very controversial topic. She told me this surgery is a very big surgery and you might have to stay out of work for a while. It'll take you a lot, so you probably don't have to worry about it. I was a little bit surprised to hear that because, whether the treatment protocol is invasive or not, that doesn't matter. As long as I need a treatment protocol, I have to get it right. I told her that, at least what you can do is refer me to Dr. Schnittger's office or Dr. Schnittger's clinic, and that she did. Then I got into Dr. Schnittger's clinic. Dr. Schnittger, as you know, has a very busy clinic and everywhere from US, people come here with myocardial bridge. Luckily, since I was already on Stanford system, it was very easy and quick for me to get their attention, but the scheduler called me and said, that was end of August, she said, we don't have any availability until November.

By that time the ER became almost like my second home. Every now and then I was having these chest pains and although they did not tell from the hospital, they said that you don't have any obstructive disease. They still gave me nitroglycerin, of course, longer acting nitroglycerine. They said if you take one nitroglycerine after chest pain, you take two, three, and if it doesn't go away after three, you have to come back to the ER. Since then, since August till the surgery, ER became my second home.

In fact, I have been to ER so many times that there are certain physicians that I actually got in repeat. There was one time I went there, I saw one doctor, and then a few weeks later I went there. She was there again on that same day, and she said, oh, I recognize you from a few weeks ago. This was my story. I kept on going, so after learning that I won't be able to get into surgery until November, I used my Stanford alumni email address to email to Dr. Schnittger directly and asked her, hey, I was a student here, so as an alumnus, would you consider squeezing me in earlier? She was able to get me into her office sooner than November. In September, there was another cancellation and I was able to see her for the first time.

JH: One thing she does say, and to your point, you're a young man and the longer this goes, especially if you have a cholesterol issue, 100% of the myocardial bridges have occlusion or narrowing where the artery enters into the heart. Everyone. The longer it goes, the worse it gets. It's not going to get better by delaying it.

Raisul Islam: No, it won't. And even my cholesterol was kept under control with medications very aggressively. Still, I had plaque at the entrance of the myocardial bridge. I got myself in the first time and by that time she saw all my results, the cath, the CT and angiogram and everything. The first time I went there she actually got all the images in her phone and showed to me, here is where we think is the bridge, here. See the cath? This moment there is the artery getting vanished for a few seconds. You slow down the frames, that's where it's getting, pressed by the muscle. This is the first time she said your pain is very real and it's being caused by the ischemia because of the myocardial bridge. She initially said that the surgery is definitely a big one, so we are going to try the medications first. She said that you already had a cath, although it's not a provocative cath with all the measurements and everything, but I am convinced that you will need this treatment. She started me on this nebivolol that she actually prefers, this is a beta blocker, but it had some other effect of increasing the release of the nitric oxide inside the artery. That's the first step. All the steps, this type of first medication, and then the invasive test. It's basically the standard of care for her clinic. I think you also know about that. I started taking the medication and it did not really solve any problem.

Then, it felt like a house of cards. It started by November; I was almost disabled. In fact, I had to ask to my primary care physician to issue a disability placard for me, because I wasn't able to walk, I wasn't able to get up the stairs. Every time I go up the stairs in my home, I get palpitations. I get chest tightness. I am short of breath. I have two dogs and I could not take them to walk. In fact, one time it happened that I went in the neighborhood with my dog and in the middle of walking I had to call my wife. Hey, you need to pick me up because it's too much. She's the one I have always been trying to push through or ignoring this kind of pain. Dr. Schnittger told me in our first visit that there is no powering through a chest pain. If you have chest pain, whatever you are doing, you have to stop. You have to stop because you are causing more harm to your heart if you are pushing through chest pain.

JH: So many of us did exactly that because we're in disbelief or denial, this can't be happening. Right? No, I'm good. That's something else. It can't be my heart. I'm too young, I'm too this, I'm too that, too fit, whatever. And it comes out in every conversation we're having here. The acceptance of the reality of this is it can't be, it can't be happening to me.

Raisul Islam: I was in denial for many, many months, maybe even years. Right? So finally, I told her that the medication is not working, and I was referred to Dr. Jennifer Tremmel, who does the provocative cath. I had my cath early December. I had my provocative cath and she did all sorts of dobutamine (a medication used to speed the heart up) and she checked for endothelial dysfunction. Finally, we got a quantification of the myocardial bridge. It was six centimeters long. One millimeter deep. This is towards the deeper end. It's very long. It's six centimeters long and there is severe endothelial dysfunction which causes the vasospasm. I have the whole shebang.

At the follow-up visit, Dr. Schnittger told me that times, she seemed to be very positive about the surgery because she said I think you will see a lot of improvement in your life. By that time, I was kind of scared. Not only scared, but also worried about what would happen. I have a daughter, there are two dogs. It's going to be very difficult for my wife to take care of all of them. I was a little bit worried. But she seems to be pushing me. We spent about an hour and she said all the things, she answered very meticulously about everything, every detail about the surgery and everything. Then I was referred to Dr. Jack Boyd and I saw Dr. Boyd on January 23rd to have a surgery on the 24th.

JH: Which is very quick, relatively speaking.

Raisul Islam: Yes. And I feel extremely lucky that it took me a relatively short period of time to get into the bridge clinic, most importantly, that we all, the myocardial bridge patients, go through this sort of disbelief or sort of people around them, or the doctors actually do not want to believe them. For my case, it was probably the least because I was always in the Stanford system. All the cardiologists, at least they know what it is.

JH: In fact, they tell you that as a regular patient in the hospital so frequently in the emergency room, they said, we have got to do something for the poor guy. He's probably costing us a fortune in just the emergency room. Right? So that was January 24th? We're talking to you in April. We're not even four months out from your surgery. You look amazingly healthy. You're just to the point now where you can start to lift a little bit, correct?

Raisul Islam: Yes. I am wonderful. I started a few weeks ago, but I don't think I can lift very heavy stuff. It's probably 20, 30 pounds for a short period of time. It's fine with keeping my posture and everything, but if I have to do an awkward stretch with heavy stuff, probably won't be able to do it. I still do get muscle pains. Pain in the joint. And then every incision, if the incision is really big, a lot of nerves basically are cut open. You get all sorts of fancy feeling on the incision side. Those are all there, but I am much better than any point in the last one year or more than a year. Most importantly, besides the chest pain, the fatigue that I was always talking about is gone. In fact, now that it's gone, I can realize or appreciate even more that, wow, I was in so much fatigue and I was able to do whatever I did in those last three years. I could not do much, but I still was able to do a few things. I was able to do that, and I feel like, wow, I could do that even after feeling that bad. Now, I feel a little new normal. It seems like the surgery actually created a new normal for me, which I have not felt for a long time.

JH: Let me ask you something. If there was one thing that you would like to leave those who are learning the story of your imperfect heart, what would you say?

Raisul Islam: There is no powering through a chest pain. You should keep looking for answers. If you have a chest pain that you do not know what's the origin, you should know what is the origin. It might not be cardiac related in the end, but whatever it is, you should take care of it and always listen to your body. I think all these signs and symptoms that your body is producing, it's telling you that something is not right. Not everything is in your mind. I have been telling that myself about my fatigue, that maybe I'm just too tired, maybe. It's all in my mind. Maybe I have become more lethargic these days. I'm not. I'm not as active anymore, that's the last thing that I want to tell everyone. I think the doctors also need to listen to their patients.

KELLY PORTILLO: The Intersection of Fact and Faith

(How her faith became the foundation of support for a positive outcome to surgery.)

At just 13, Kelly was a vibrant teenager in a karate class when her life took an unexpected turn. During a routine session, her heart raced abnormally fast, accompanied by chest pain akin to a heart attack. Rushed to the ER, doctors dismissed her symptoms as anxiety, despite Kelly feeling mentally well. Over the years, her condition worsened—simple activities like running or snowboarding became insurmountable as she endured frequent episodes of chest pain and rapid heartbeat. After high school, these episodes escalated, leading to a diagnosis of Supraventricular Tachycardia (SVT-a rapid heart rate) and her first heart ablation at 19. Though the procedure promised a high success rate, it failed, leaving her reliant on medication. Subsequent ablations also failed, with the risk of severe complications halting further interventions. Kelly's journey became one of resilience, navigating uncertainty and fear as she faced a relentless heart condition.

This was Kelly's story so far—a story of misdiagnoses, dismissals, failed procedures, and relentless struggle. However, it was also a tale of resilience, a testament to a young woman's unwavering determination to seek answers and reclaim her life. That reclamation required an incredible amount of faith to bring it to a conclusion.

Jeff Holden (Host): Kelly, yours is a most interesting story, and I'm going to have you start, if you could, from that karate class when you were 13 years old where you noticed something was up.

Kelly Portillo (Guest): Yes, in my karate class, which I had been taking for about six months, I was actually getting ready to spar, so I was sitting down on the ground when my heart started beating fast and that was abnormal. I never felt that before and I started getting chest pain and it felt like a heart attack. Even though I was only 13, I kind of knew what a heart attack symptom was, I was having chest pain down my arm and felt really lightheaded and I just sat on the sidelines for a couple of minutes and my symptoms didn't go away. We ended up calling my mom and my mom took me to the ER to get checked out. At the ER the doctor just ran the EKG, no other tests and said oh, you just have anxiety. You're 13 years old. You can't possibly have a heart attack. I was led to believe that it was just in my head and I was having anxiety, even though mentally I felt well.

JH: That's scary for a 13-year-old kid. As you grew 13, 14, 15, these things kept occurring, right?

Kelly Portillo: Right, as I got older, I was having more episodes of my symptoms, of my heart rate beating really fast and I was getting bad chest pain. I was in junior high at the time and we had to run the mile in P.E. class and I couldn't do it. I thought, oh well, I'm just out of shape and I have anxiety. I just became embarrassed about my symptoms, because that's a mental problem, not a physical problem.

JH: I'll bet you were probably thinking to yourself what's wrong with me? Why am I like this? Those are really formative years, your self-esteem is being built and your confidence is being built, and here you are struggling just to maintain.

Kelly Portillo: Yes, it was almost unbearable. I let myself become really shy and not wanting to talk to anybody because I didn't want to explain how I really felt. All my friends were running around and enjoying life and I had these symptoms. The doctor said, oh, you just have anxiety. I didn't know what to make of that. At 13, 14, 15 years old I tried to do activities, tried surfing, snowboarding. I was able to do that a little bit, but it was always such a struggle. I was embarrassed that I couldn't keep up with the other kids my age.

JH: You become exhausted, experience shortness of breath, chest pains, even with exertion.

Kelly Portillo: Yes.

JH: Somehow, you get through high school with these symptoms that you're still thinking are mentally originated as opposed to physically originated, what happens next? How do we go into young adulthood after you graduate?

Kelly Portillo: After I graduated, the episodes became more frequent and I was having, probably twice a week, the fast heart rate and chest pain and I was short of breath all the time at that point. I would have these episodes where my heart rate would go really, really high and you could actually see my shirt moving because my heart would beat so fast. I tried to take ibuprofen and rest, as the doctor would say go decompress for your anxiety. I tried to do that and it was just getting harder and harder to live.

Finally, one day, I got the episode again, I was at my aunt's house. She was making dinner, I was helping, and I got a bad episode. My parents eventually took me to the ER because it felt like I was going to pass out at that point. At the ER, they took my vital signs. My heart rate was 190. Then they gave me an EKG and said you have SVT (supraventricular tachycardia—a faster-than-normal heart rate). Okay! I have a real heart problem. We dealt with that. They said, if it happens again, just come back, but to follow up with a cardiologist. I followed up with a cardiologist and they suggested that I could do an ablation, which would be 95% successful if I did that. I agreed that it's just a procedure. I agreed to have my heart ablated when I was 19 years old.

JH: And so that was your first ablation for ventricular tachycardia, and in the process between 13 and 19, were you on any other medication other than just Tylenol or aspirin or anything like that?

Kelly Portillo: Well, at about 13 to like 15 years old, I was on anxiety medicine that a doctor prescribed. It actually made me feel worse. It made me feel lightheaded, and I got more chest pain. My symptoms were worse. It wasn't even helping my anxiety. I decided that I didn't want to take anxiety medicine, but other than that I was not on any medication.

JH: At 19 or so you have the ablation. What happens next?

Kelly Portillo: I had the ablation. You stay overnight when you have one done. The next day my heart rate was fast all the time. It was about 140, just resting in the bed. My doctor reassured me that sometimes that happens with ablations, that things are opened up now and the blood flow is going through your heart, that should go away in a couple of months. But in a couple of months, I still continued to have a fast heart rate all the time. They decided to put me on metoprolol (which treats high blood pressure and chest pain) and that helped some. I still continue to have a fast heart rate of 140 resting and when I would exercise it would go maybe 180, 190.

JH: What happens next?

Kelly Portillo: I got referred to a different electrophysiologist and he suggested that I had a different arrhythmia, not SVT this time. He thought it was something called sinus tachycardia, that he was sure that if he ablated that area my symptoms could go away. I was about 20 years old at that time.

I agreed to have the second ablation for this second arrhythmia. I had that and the next day, I was in the hospital, and my heart rate was still the same. It was about 140 resting, 180 walking around and the doctor said well, that ablation didn't work, we could do a third ablation. I could try to ablate the areas that I think are causing the problem. I agreed to have the third ablation about two months afterward. The third ablation lasted six hours and he gave up and said my heart's beating fast and I'm not sure exactly where this is coming from. He wanted to ablate my SA node, but my frantic nerve was in the way. He said that he couldn't do that because if he ablated the frantic nerve, I would have my diaphragm paralyzed for life and I would be short of breath even more, forever. He didn't want to put that risk on me and I didn't want that either, so we left it at that for now.

JH: After the third ablation, I'm sure you're still on the metoprolol and trying to maintain, but nothing's really changed for the better. You're 21-ish years old. What happens between then and the next few years?

Kelly Portillo: At about 21, I was on 200 milligrams of metoprolol a day. I basically tried every medication there was to control the heart rate and chest pain. Nothing was helping. I was maxed out and my quality of life was very poor. I couldn't go out with friends, I couldn't go to college, I couldn't do normal life things. My doctor felt bad and said we could do a thoracotomy ablation where I could move the frantic nerve and see if we could ablate the SA node and see if they could calm down the fast heart rate.

I was so desperate. I was almost bedridden. I couldn't go out. My dad had to do different things for me, and I felt like this is not a life that I want to live. I agreed to have the thoracotomy procedure, even though later down the road my doctor told me that was the first time they've ever done it. They just made up that surgery and procedure. When I was 22, I had that procedure. It was super painful. I burst an artery in my chest. I almost didn't make it. I was in the ICU. I thought I was going to die because I was bleeding out from my chest tube and thankfully, they were able to give me a second surgery and save me. After that my heart rate did get better. I was still on medication, but something was still not right. I was still having chest pain and shortness of breath.

JH: You were a guinea pig for them to practice the procedure on?

Kelly Portillo: Right.

JH: And you didn't improve significantly. Maybe the heart rate came down, but the experience of symptoms didn't go away. What was the reaction? What did they say?

Kelly Portillo: They said that I just had to live like that. I was out of options. They didn't know what was wrong. They would always tell me there's something bigger going on, but we don't know what. I would just have to live like that. I was in my early 20s and pretty upset. That was my life, but I accepted it because there was nothing I could do. Different doctors I went to, they all said the same thing, they don't know. They said I think you're just born with an arrhythmic gentry heart. That's what they called it. There's no explanation, that's just you.

JH: Lucky you, right?

Kelly Portillo: Right.

JH: Somewhere in that time frame you make a decision to say this isn't working for me and I'm going to do something differently about it after four ablations. I think at some point something else happened too, where they put a pacemaker in.

Kelly Portillo: Yes, a pacemaker, because shortly after the thoracotomy I started having symptoms that I was going to pass out. I got a Holter monitor put on and they said that I was having three-second pauses often.

They ablated my SA (sinus) node too much, and so now my heart was pausing and going too low, so their suggestion was to put a pacemaker in me so my heart wouldn't just stop.

JH: How old were you at the pacemaker stage?

Kelly Portillo: 23 years old.

JH: What was it that caused you to say there's more here, I've got to find something? How did you go about doing that?

Kelly Portillo: Well, after the pacemaker I felt a little bit better, but I knew there was still something wrong. A couple of years later I got another arrhythmia, AFib. That's so many arrhythmias. I was like this doesn't seem right. I had another ablation for the AFib. I still continued to have frequent episodes of chest pain, shortness of breath, fast heart rate, even after all these ablations and different medications and procedures. Then my insurance changed. I had to go to a different doctor, and I told them hey, look, I'm having really bad chest pain. It's going down my arm. I feel like I'm having a heart attack. Please, if there's anything that you can do, let's do it. I've had a treadmill test and echocardiogram, but they said that it was normal. My doctor finally said since you're having all these symptoms, let's try to do a CT angiogram, a test that I've never had before. I had the CT angiogram and it showed a deep 25-millimeter myocardial bridge that went through the right ventricle. Great! I have the solution. But the doctor who did the test said oh, those are benign, that's a benign condition. We don't treat those. That's not the cause of your symptoms. Then, he even said everyone has that, it's not a big deal. As I did my own research on myocardial bridges, which I'd never heard of before, I came upon Stanford's website, and I was looking at all the symptoms and at every single one of those symptoms. I didn't think it was right that he said that was benign when I have every symptom of that heart defect.

JH: The one thing he did right at least, was he did the CT scan to identify what might be going on. The unfortunate part is, while he discovers it, he dismisses it. And he was close on the other thing. Not everybody has one, but about a quarter of the population has one, and this is part of the process every one of us who goes through the discovery of the myocardial bridge goes through: where people dismiss it, calling it benign. It doesn't cause symptoms, yet they can't identify what's wrong with us. For people who are symptomatic, it's easy for us to say obviously, that's the only logical explanation of something that's different, especially in your case, with the ablations, the pacemaker, the SA node, there's nothing left to do. Yet you're still symptomatic. The good news is you find Stanford. About what time was that? What year? How old were you at that point?

Kelly Portillo: I was 31 years old.

JH: Okay. You went through a period of about eight years there where you just had to deal with the symptoms.

Kelly Portillo: Yes, I had to deal with the symptoms for about eight years. It was getting hard for me to work. I work in a hospital, in the pre-op unit, and I could barely do that. I would come home and had no quality of life, just so tired, so much pain. My friend even offered to make me food every day because I couldn't even do that. It was getting worse and worse as I got older.

JH: Well, it's a great friend who's willing to help you to that degree, that's for sure.

Kelly Portillo: Yeah, she also works. She's a nurse and works in the hospital with me.

JH: You get the connection to Stanford. Things are starting to look up a little bit because you now realize I've got this thing and this thing matches their diagnosis, their process. What is the next step? I know you had a little stumbling block in there as well when you were pursuing Stanford—and that was your insurance company, correct?

Kelly Portillo: Right. I convinced my cardiologist to give me a referral to Stanford, even though he's like, well, go ahead and do it, but the surgery is big. I don't think you should do it. It's probably not even going to help you. I did get the referral, and my insurance did approve me for one visit. But at the last minute they said, oh, it's denied because it's not in network. I was so close to talking with Dr. Schnittger. I said I'm going to pay for the appointment because I don't want to miss it. And there happened to be a cancellation. I got to talk to Dr. Schnittger within three weeks of booking that appointment and I didn't want to miss that.

I saw Dr. Schnittger via a video appointment and she was pretty convinced that this bridge was the source of all my symptoms since I was 13. I had tried every medication at that point. She didn't want to go that route of trying different medications. She said if you were a candidate for the surgery, we would need a provocative heart cath. I would like you to come over to Stanford and get one of those. I said, okay, great. When we went to ask for authorization for the heart cath, my insurance did indeed deny me for that because it was out of network.

JH: You did take that bull by the horns yourself and I think it's important for people to hear what you did. You're in the state of California, you're in Southern California, for anybody who is in the state of California, this is a process that can be done. I don't know about other states, but if you're similar to the insurance process in California, this may work as well. Share with us what you did, Kelly.

Kelly Portillo: Through my insurance, I appealed several times, and they kept denying me and wanted me to go to in network doctors that they thought that could do the unroofing. When I actually called the doctor, they didn't even know how to spell myocardial bridge. They had no idea. I did do what they said and went to the different cardiac surgeons and electrophysiologists and cardiologists. There's a process in California that's called Department of Managed Healthcare. If your insurance denies you and you feel like you have a true medical problem, you can apply to them and if they approve you, they overturn what the insurance says. Even if the insurance says no, if the Department of Managed Healthcare approves you, then they have to cover everything. I did that. It took me almost a year to get through that whole process and it was a lot. Eventually, the Department of Managed Healthcare approved me for full coverage, 100% for that.

JH: Congratulations! That is such a great story to hear that you got through that first hurdle. It was a year since you had the conversation with Dr. Schnittger, but to get to the provocative test you had to go through this years' worth of insurance grief. But you finally got there.

Kelly Portillo: Right.

JH: Now you've got the opportunity to get in and get your provocative test. What happens next?

Kelly Portillo: I had the heart cath and Dr. Schnittger—I remember lying in the cath lab room—and she said, your test showed that you are 40% compressed on your LAD (left anterior descending artery) at rest and you're about 80% compressed with exercise. You would be a great candidate for unroofing surgery. I just couldn't believe that I actually had a diagnosis and a solution. I was just sitting in the cath lab looking up at the ceiling like, is this really real? Could I get better from this 25 years of pain and suffering? Dr. Schnittger was so confident that I could benefit from this surgery.

JH: I think your determination and perseverance through so many outside struggles, on top of the diagnosis and the process that you went through really made a difference. Now it's time to get to Stanford. Share with us what happened then.

Kelly Portillo: Well, after my heart cath, a couple of days later, I was scheduled for the surgery. About three days later I went back, and my best friend was supposed to go with me to the surgery but at the last minute she got sick, so I didn't have anyone else to go with me. My dad was going to meet me after the surgery, but I didn't want to cancel because a lot of money was spent on my flights and my Airbnb, so I decided to go by myself to the surgery and go out and let my faith and trust be in God. He has brought me through this for 25 years. Why would He leave me now? I went out on faith, and I went to the surgery by myself.

JH: If I'm not mistaken, there was an interesting situation on the plane on the way out.

Kelly Portillo: Yes. I flew into San Jose and the wheels of the plane were touching down in San Jose. I got this sinking feeling like oh, wow, I'm here in a place that I've only been just a couple of days ago and about to have the biggest surgery a person could have and I'm by myself. I started sweating and getting so much anxiety. I don't think I can do this. I know there's a lot of money spent, but I don't think I can do this by myself. Also, the thought that Stanford puts catheters, pain catheters in the day before surgery. They told me I can't get sedation because I don't have anybody with me.

All these fears came into my head. I was just shaking. I was like, okay, I've got to do this, even though it was really hard. I stood up out of the plane seat, I looked to my left and on the guy across from me, his arm was tattooed. "I could do all things through Christ, who strengthens me." At that point I knew that I'm doing this. I'm not alone, I'm alone, but yet not alone. After that I was like, okay, I'm okay, I'm going to do this.

JH: Good for you and that's awesome! We have a gentleman that we interviewed for another program that we produce and his line was, "do your best, let God do the rest", and you absolutely did your best. You got yourself there. Now you're there, you're going to go through the process at Stanford and your surgery was in August of 2022, correct?

Kelly Portillo: Correct.

JH: Tell us a little about the process and where your head was at going in and coming out, and then we'll get to how you are today.

Kelly Portillo: Going in I was a little scared. I had the pain catheters put in without sedation, so that was a bit hard, but my faith was in the Lord. I knew that I just had a trust in him. Going into the surgery I did that and I felt like, okay, I'm not alone in this. I went into that morning of surgery and the staff is great at Stanford. I am a big Star Wars fan, so they were talking to me about that. They wanted me to do Chewbacca voices as I go under anesthesia. Then the nurse even held my hand. She knew I was by myself in the operating room and the OR nurse held my hand while I went to sleep. I woke up in the ICU. I was not intubated and right when I woke up, I felt like a weight had been lifted off my chest. I felt like light as a feather, which I never felt that way ever. I thought maybe it's, maybe too much pain medicine. But no, it was different. I was able to talk. I wasn't even in pain. I called my friend that night and my roommate was supposed to come with me and she's like, your voice is really different. You sound totally different than how you were, like you had this little spunk in your voice even though you just had open heart surgery a couple of hours before. I knew I was healed.

JH: Well, I can even see as you're telling the story, you're smiling. You can just see it all comes back. The revelation that you're better, something's changed and that's amazing to see. You are post-surgery and, before I get there let me ask you about endothelial dysfunction. Do you know where you stood on that?

Kelly Portillo: I was tested as moderate.

JH: This means something to those of us who were diagnosed with *severe* endothelial dysfunction. It's another symptom that over time, you probably would have gotten to where it just deteriorated, and the artery just got more and more broken down to where it really began to function improperly. Even though it took 20 plus years, at least you got it when you were still relatively young. You got through the surgery well. I assume your dad made it up there post-surgery at some point?

Kelly Portillo: Yes, the day after surgery he made it there.

JH: Great, so you had somebody with you afterwards. How long did it take you before you actually realized that what you felt post-surgery immediately was real and something had changed for the better, for good?

Kelly Portillo: It was a day after they got you up to walk. I walked around the nurse's station. I had no chest pain. The last time I had chest pain was the morning before the surgery. I walked around the nurse's station with no symptoms, so it was very soon after that I knew it's different, that I'm cured.

JH: You almost have to pinch yourself and say is this really happening?

Kelly Portillo: It didn't feel real and I was like, well, if I feel this good the day after, how well am I going to feel in a week or two? I continued to get better and better. I was walking fast. The physical therapist at the hospital said wow, you walk really fast for just having had open-heart surgery. I'm usually walking really slowly and have chest pain.

JH: Today, more than a year-and-a-half later, what have you noticed differently about your physical capability?

Kelly Portillo: I no longer have chest pain, I no longer have shortness of breath. I walk for miles at a time and I got a bike, so I'm riding a bike. Those thoughts never came into my head before, never exercised. I avoided all that. Now I want to do that. Now I'm looking for things like okay, next year, I want to go snowboarding, or this summer I'm going to go surfing. It just continues to get better. Actually, at my nine-month recovery mark, I had an opportunity to go to Israel with my church and I got the blessing from Dr. Boyd. He actually wanted me to go, and we went into Jordan and Petra. I did a five-mile hike without a problem. I could never have done that before.

JH: How cool is that? What an experience for anybody. And especially an experience for somebody who, just a little over a year earlier, was unable to walk a block.

Kelly Portillo: Right, it was. I walked all over Israel for 15 days and didn't have a problem. It was unbelievable.

JH: What would you say, if you look back, really helped you get through this entire process, from the uncertainty, the pain and the frustration in your twenties, which lasted eight, 10 years till you finally realized I've got this thing called a bridge and I've got to do something about it? What did you lean on most? For those people who are also in a similar situation going, "I've got this problem, I don't know what it is, I'm working through it," what can you tell them?

Kelly Portillo: It's my faith in the Lord. When I was 15, I became a Christian and that's my firm foundation, my rock. I've learned in life anything can happen. Things change. My symptoms changed. What didn't change is the Lord. He was there with me the whole time. I really would just pray because it was so uncertain. Doctors could even tell me my future. But I knew I had a future with the Lord, like no matter what, even if I passed away from these conditions, that I would go to heaven because

I put my faith in the Lord Jesus and that's who I rely on. My family and friends are great, but the Lord is always there. He doesn't change. He's the same today, yesterday and forever.

JH: I think that's so important for so many people who are struggling, and I know everybody's belief could be a little bit different, but it's a belief in a higher power to some degree, that if you have that support, it helps you get through these challenges. So many of the people that we've spoken with on the program have said something to that effect. They had a belief, whether it was a higher power, if it was Christ, or how they perceived it, a God. Whatever it was, there was something beyond them that they were able to rely on and lean on to support them through the challenges, especially the anxiety, frustration, fear of surgery. When you were going into surgery, do you remember, literally as they were wheeling you in, what you were thinking?

Kelly Portillo: Yes, I was thinking okay, no matter what happens, the Lord has me and I'm going to be okay.

JH: When you were in the ICU, what was going through your head? Now you were a bit drugged up, but you sensed something was different. What were you thinking at that point?

Kelly Portillo: I was thinking, well, is this really true? That I feel this good? I expected the worst. I think I have a high pain tolerance, but I really don't. I've been there a lot, so it takes a lot of pain medicine to calm me down. I felt so good that it was like, is this really real? I was determined just to recover well and do what the doctor says and take one day at a time.

JH: Then, you have your sternotomy. You're a year and a half out now, so you would know if there were any issues. You've been okay. No issues, no sternal pain, everything healed up properly?

Kelly Portillo: Yes.

JH: Good for you because we've had five women on my podcast, "Imperfect Heart," to date and three of them have had sternal issues.

Kelly Portillo: I don't have anything.

JH: That's wonderful. It doesn't appear that this is a common occurrence. I know it's not. It just happened to be that three of our people had it, so it looks like the percentages are slightly against smaller women that you're going to have issues. I think we'll accumulate some success stories of perfect healing. So, things are good? Work is good? You're still at the same hospital, right?

Kelly Portillo: Right, for 14 years now.

JH: Amazing. That's fantastic to hear. I know if I don't ask this question, everybody's going to be wondering why. Do you still have the pacemaker?

Kelly Portillo: I do. I will have that pacemaker for life. My heart is now 100% reliant on it because they say your heart gets lazy when it has something to beat for it. I'll have that for life and it doesn't bother me. I forget I have it. I just get it checked every six months or so.

JH: The pacemaker really is just there for the benefit now of anything that should be aberrant in an arrhythmia which, if I'm not mistaken when we were talking earlier, you've had no episodes of arrhythmia since the surgery.

Kelly Portillo: Right, I had my pacemaker checked maybe four or five times since surgery and I've had zero arrhythmias. I would have 3,000 a month before surgery.

JH: Have you shared any of this with the doctor that originally prescribed or diagnosed the myocardial bridge?

Kelly Portillo: Yes, I did tell him because I happen to work with him at the hospital. He sees me all the time and he's like how are you doing? Did you go to Stanford? I said, yes, I did, and all my symptoms were gone. I told him that and he's like, well, you look really good. Wow, that really helped. I'm starting to believe that this is a problem.

My electrophysiologist is so amazed at my recovery and is like wow, all these years I had so many problems and all of a sudden, I'm completely fine. The process they did, they've changed it because of me. If anyone has a symptom of myocardial bridge, they will be referred without hesitation to Stanford and get the treatment that they need. I'm quite happy for others in my situation.

JH: If you were being asked, somebody says geez Kelly, I've got the same situation. I'm really anxious about it. I'm not sure if I should get the surgery. I'm just starting this process. I know you went through 20-plus years and I'm in the same boat. I don't know if I'm going to find out fast enough. What would you say to somebody who's just beginning that journey, who now realizes they have a myocardial bridge?

Kelly Portillo: I would tell them to be an advocate for themselves. Even though the doctor may say like, oh, you have a bridge, but it's not the cause of your symptoms. I would just go and push and ask for the necessary tests, ask for the referrals and don't give up. There are times where the days are long and you're in pain and you don't know what to do. You want to give up on life. Don't give up. I never thought that I would get better, but in an instant I was better. If people can hold on to that hope, just be patient and get the test done, there can be a solution for you. Whether it's medication or actual surgery, there is hope and we should never give up.

CHAPTER SIX

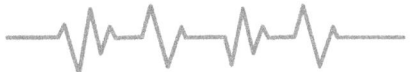

What Would You Find If You Spoke With A Genius?

(My Conversation with Open AI's Chat GPT.)

THE CHAPTER THAT FOLLOWS IS ONE THAT I THOUGHT NEEDED TO BE explained. When we first learn of our condition, or we get some understanding that our heart has this thing called a myocardial bridge, we can't ask enough questions. We can't get to Google or Chat GPT soon enough to find out what the heck this condition is. In many cases, that's all we have to go on. What is it with those two words: myocardial bridge? What's that? You're far enough along in the book to know that it's likely you're not going to get a proper answer the first few times around. For the podcast, I thought it would make for quite a conversation to interview the internet. What would it look like if I asked the questions we all ask when we learn of our condition? What is it we say when we first hear those two words, myocardial bridge, mentioned in some context relative to our symptoms? I did what any of us would do or have done, I started a conversation online with a bot. I reached out to Open AI's Chat GPT and just started firing away. Quite remarkably, the conversation was biased toward bridges being symptomatic. Maybe that was me and the way I asked the questions, but it was encouraging to see that I didn't get dismissed. I didn't get gaslit. I got answers based on the vast knowledge that's available to the crawlers and search engines and bots and it came back with answers that coincide with what we all know. Myocardial bridges are symptomatic and they can be the cause of sudden cardiac death. I was quite blown away with how the conversation transpired. You might say I got a little carried away, but it was going so well, I just couldn't control myself, so I kept asking more questions! I was awed. If only the medical community recognized the condition the way the bots did on Chat GPT.

What I then did after I cleaned up the responses in print, was I added some "character" to do what I could to "humanize" the interaction. It didn't come out perfectly when I translated the content to an AI voice, but what was produced is a podcast episode that is tremendously informative and tutorial. The chapter that follows is assembled in a class like outline that I hope gives you enough information to do what you need to do in your own best interest. I even asked how to dismiss a doctor that is not giving you what you need. I know that can be difficult for some of us. We tend to be too *nice*. We can't be too *nice* when we're advocating for our own well-being, in this case, it could be for our very own lives. Please take the chapter as it's meant to be. It is not the end all be all answer to everything. It is a bit entertaining when you get down to it, and it is full of great content, support and actionable items for you to be the very best steward of your own health.

Let me introduce you to my genius guest, Chaddy Gpt.

Jeff Holden (Host): Chaddy Gpt, welcome to Imperfect Heart.

Chaddy Gpt (Guest): Thank you Jeff, it's a pleasure to be here. I just love what you're doing for those with myocardial bridges and the Imperfect Heart Community.

JH: Let me ask, are you aware of myocardial bridges and their consequences?

Chaddy Gpt: Yes, a **myocardial bridge** is a congenital heart condition where a coronary artery, instead of lying on the surface of the heart as it normally does, tunnels through the heart muscle or myocardium as it's known. This causes the artery to be "bridged" by the muscle.

During the heart's contraction, Systole, the bridged artery can become compressed, potentially reducing blood flow to the heart muscle. While many people with myocardial bridges are asymptomatic and never require treatment, others might experience symptoms such as:

- **Chest pain or angina**
- **Shortness of breath**
- **Palpitations**
- **Fatigue**
- **Radiating pain in the arm, neck or jaw**

In severe cases, myocardial bridges may contribute to conditions such as myocardial ischemia or even arrhythmias.

Myocardial bridges are often detected through imaging studies like:

- **Coronary angiography**
- **CT angiography**
- **Intravascular ultrasound (IVUS)**
- **Stress testing** to assess its functional impact.
- **Provocative testing to invasively identify as much about that bridge as possible**

Management depends on the severity of the symptoms:

1. **Lifestyle Changes**: Avoiding triggers that increase heart rate or stress on the heart.
2. **Medications**: Beta-blockers or calcium channel blockers may be used to reduce heart rate and myocardial oxygen demand.
3. **Surgical Interventions**:
    - Myotomy or surgical cutting of the myocardial bridge, more commonly known as "unroofing" surgery.
    - In some cases, coronary artery bypass grafting (CABG) may be considered.
4. **Stents** should be avoided due to risks in the dynamic compression zone.

JH: Why is it, do you think, so many cardiologists dismiss myocardial bridges when the patient is symptomatic?

Chaddy Gpt: Sure. The dismissal of **myocardial bridges** by some cardiologists, even when patients are symptomatic, may be due to a combination of factors related to medical training, perception of the condition, and diagnostic limitations:

First, They're Historically Considered Benign

- For decades, myocardial bridges were thought to be largely benign anomalies with little clinical significance. Many cardiologists were trained under the assumption that MBs rarely cause significant symptoms.
- Since the majority of people with MBs are asymptomatic, there is a tendency to generalize this to all cases.

Second, Inconsistent Symptoms and Diagnostic Challenges

- **Symptoms Mimic Other Conditions:** For example, chest pain, palpitations, and shortness of breath are non-specific and often attributed to more common issues like anxiety, musculoskeletal pain, or non-cardiac causes.
- **Dynamic Nature:** MBs compress the artery during systole, making the impact difficult to detect in standard tests like resting angiograms. Specialized tests, like stress imaging or intravascular ultrasound (IVUS), may not always be ordered or available.
- **Underappreciated in Testing:** Some diagnostic tools fail to fully capture the functional significance of the compression, leading to false reassurance from "normal" results.

Third, Focus on Structural Heart Disease

- **Shift in Focus:** Many cardiologists prioritize conditions with clear, immediate structural or obstructive pathologies, like coronary artery disease, over dynamic conditions like MBs.
- **Lack of Emphasis in Guidelines:** MBs have not been widely emphasized in cardiovascular guidelines, so treatment pathways can seem less standardized or urgent.

Fourth, Bias Toward More Common Diagnoses

- **Cognitive Bias:** Physicians may focus on more prevalent conditions (e.g., atherosclerosis) and dismiss MBs as an incidental finding rather than the root cause.
- **Diagnostic Fatigue:** Patients with vague or persistent symptoms might face skepticism if a cause isn't immediately apparent, leading to frustration for both patient and physician.

Fifth, Limited Awareness of Advanced Insights

- Recent studies have highlighted MBs as a potential cause of **ischemia, arrhythmias, and even sudden cardiac events.** However, not all clinicians stay updated with evolving research or have access to the latest diagnostic tools.
- **Knowledge Gaps:** Some physicians may lack experience with managing symptomatic MBs or may not recognize the need for multidisciplinary approaches (e.g., collaboration with specialized imaging cardiologists or surgeons).

Sixth, Complex Management and Patient Advocacy

- **Reluctance to Intervene:** Treatments like surgery or medications for MBs are often seen as invasive or unnecessary, especially when the risks seem to outweigh benefits in mild cases.
- **Patient Advocacy Challenges:** Patients may need to persistently advocate for themselves to have their symptoms and concerns taken seriously.

Seeking a second opinion from a cardiologist with expertise in **coronary anomalies** or **microvascular dysfunction** may provide more clarity and appropriate management.

JH: Chaddy, it's my opinion and that of many cardiologists I've spoken with, that you can you die from the effects of a myocardial bridge. If not directly, at the very least, indirectly. Would you agree that a myocardial bridge could be the cause of sudden cardiac death?

Chaddy Gpt: Absolutely, while most people with a **myocardial bridge** live normal lives without significant complications, in rare cases, it can lead to serious or even fatal outcomes. The risk largely depends on the severity of the bridge, its location, and the extent of compression during systole. In my opinion, here's how a myocardial bridge could contribute to life-threatening events:

One: Myocardial Ischemia or Reduced Blood Flow

- The compression of a coronary artery by the myocardial bridge can reduce or obstruct blood flow to the heart muscle during systole, especially if the artery is significantly compressed (>50%) or the bridge affects a critical coronary artery like the **left anterior descending or LAD** artery.
- Persistent ischemia may lead to **angina, myocardial infarction, which is a heart attack**, or even sudden cardiac death.

Two: Arrhythmias

- The altered blood flow and shear stress in the coronary artery can irritate the heart's electrical system, leading to arrhythmias.
- Ventricular arrhythmias like ventricular tachycardia or fibrillation, can be life-threatening and a cause of sudden cardiac death.

Three: Coronary Artery Spasm

- MBs can provoke spasms in the coronary artery, further restricting blood flow.
- This can lead to acute ischemic events or sudden cardiac arrest.

Four: Plaque Formation or Rupture

- The turbulence and mechanical stress caused by the bridge can promote the development of atherosclerosis just proximal to the bridge. In some cases, this plaque can rupture, causing an acute blockage.
- This can result in a heart attack or sudden death.

Five: Heart Failure

- Chronic ischemia due to a myocardial bridge may weaken the heart muscle over time, potentially leading to heart failure.
- In severe cases, this may contribute to mortality.

Risk Factors for Fatal Outcomes:

- Deep or long myocardial bridges.
- Significant arterial compression (>70%).
- Bridges affecting the **proximal LAD artery** also known as the "widow-maker".
- Coexisting coronary artery disease or spasms.
- Lack of appropriate medical or surgical management.

Prevention and Management:

- **Medications:** Beta-blockers and calcium channel blockers reduce heart rate and myocardial oxygen demand, mitigating symptoms and risk.
- **Surgical Myotomy (Unroofing):** In severe cases, surgically relieving the compression may reduce the risk.
- **Lifestyle Changes:** Avoiding triggers like intense exercise, stress, and stimulants, for example, caffeine, can help reduce symptoms.
- **Regular Monitoring:** Periodic imaging and stress tests to assess progression and risk.

If you suspect or have been diagnosed with a myocardial bridge and have concerns about its severity, consulting a cardiologist with expertise in **congenital heart anomalies** or **ischemic heart disease** is crucial.

JH: That was outstanding and so much more than I expected! Chaddy, what would you say to the cardiologist who is dismissive of the symptoms, even when the patient has been diagnosed with a bridge?

Chaddy Gpt: Oh boy, I know that's a real challenge with this condition and that it can be really frustrating for the patient. Let me make these detailed suggestions for your readers. When approaching a dismissive cardiologist about symptoms related to a diagnosed myocardial bridge, it's essential to remain calm, assertive, and well-prepared. Here are some key points to communicate:

First, Acknowledge Their Expertise, but Express Concerns Clearly

Start by recognizing the cardiologist's expertise to keep the conversation constructive. Then, emphasize how the symptoms are affecting your life.

- **Example:**
  "I understand that myocardial bridges are often asymptomatic, but my symptoms—chest pain, shortness of breath, and fatigue—are significantly impacting my quality of life. I'd like to explore whether the bridge could be contributing to these issues."

Second: Reference Specific Studies or Guidelines

Mention that recent research shows myocardial bridges can cause clinically significant problems in some patients. Possibly share this book or introduce him or her to the podcast.

- **Example:**
  "I've read that myocardial bridges can sometimes lead to ischemia or arrhythmias, especially when the compression is severe or affects the LAD artery. Would additional testing like stress imaging, intravascular ultrasound or a CT angiogram help clarify this?"

Third: Highlight the Need for Further Investigation

Politely point out that dismissing the bridge without adequate evaluation could overlook potential issues.

- **Example:**
  "I'm concerned that my symptoms could be related to the bridge's functional impact. Could we consider a stress test or a second opinion to ensure nothing is missed?"

Fourth: Advocate for a Holistic Approach

Emphasize the importance of managing the symptoms and their potential impact on your health.

- **Example:**
  "Regardless of the perceived risk of the bridge, these symptoms are real and disruptive and my quality of life has diminished significantly. I'd appreciate a comprehensive plan to address them, even if it involves exploring other potential causes or consulting a specialist."

Fifth: Consider Seeking a Second Opinion

If the cardiologist remains dismissive, suggest involving another specialist without undermining their role.

- **Example:**
  "If this doesn't seem like a significant concern from your perspective, would you recommend another cardiologist or a center that specializes in coronary anomalies for a second opinion? I want to ensure we've considered all possibilities."

Sixth: Be Prepared with Documentation

Bring records of your symptoms, diagnostic tests, and any supporting research or medical articles. Presenting this information professionally can strengthen your case.

Seventh: Remain Assertive but Respectful

If you feel unheard, assert your need for further evaluation or treatment in a firm but respectful manner.

- **Example:**
  "I understand that you don't think the bridge is causing these symptoms, but I still feel that further evaluation is necessary. This is impacting my daily life, and I'd like to pursue additional testing or treatment options."

Key Message

You're advocating for your health and asking for partnership in finding answers. If the cardiologist doesn't take your concerns seriously, seeking a second opinion from a specialist familiar with myocardial bridges, for example, congenital heart disease or ischemia, is not only reasonable but sometimes essential.

JH: Wow, that's some very comprehensive guidance. Why do you think myocardial bridges are still being dismissed by medical professionals?

Chaddy Gpt: Jeff, I really think the persistent dismissal of **myocardial bridges** by some medical professionals, even when symptoms are present, can be attributed to a combination of historical perspectives, systemic challenges in medicine, and gaps in clinical understanding. Here are some key reasons:

Number one: Historical Underestimation of Clinical Significance

- **Traditional Viewpoint:** For decades, myocardial bridges were considered benign anatomical variants without significant clinical implications. This belief has been deeply ingrained in medical training.
- **Focus on Atherosclerosis:** Cardiologists are traditionally trained to focus on atherosclerotic coronary artery disease, which is more common and has clear diagnostic and treatment pathways. MBs, by contrast, have historically been viewed as incidental findings.

Number two: Lack of Standardized Guidelines

- **Absence in Major Guidelines:** Different from conditions like coronary artery disease or heart failure, myocardial bridges are not emphasized in many clinical guidelines. This leads to variability in how they are recognized and managed.
- **Diagnostic Ambiguity:** The functional significance of MBs is not always apparent on standard diagnostic tests, such as resting angiography, making it harder for clinicians to correlate symptoms with the bridge.

Number three: Diagnostic Challenges

- **Dynamic Nature of the Condition:** MB-related compression occurs during systole, which is not always evident in resting tests. Specialized tests like stress testing, intravascular ultrasound (IVUS), or fractional flow reserve (FFR) are often required, but these are not universally accessible or ordered.
- **Vague Symptoms:** Symptoms like chest pain, fatigue, or palpitations can mimic other conditions, such as anxiety or musculoskeletal issues, leading to misdiagnosis.

Number four: Bias Toward More Common Diagnoses

- **Cognitive Bias:** Physicians may gravitate toward diagnosing more common conditions, like anxiety or functional chest pain, especially if initial test results do not strongly suggest ischemia or structural abnormalities.
- **Dismissal of "Uncommon" Causes:** MBs are often dismissed as a rare cause of significant symptoms, even though they may have serious implications in some cases.

Number five: Limited Awareness of Evolving Research

- **Lag in Medical Education:** Many practicing cardiologists may not be fully aware of recent research linking myocardial bridges to conditions like myocardial ischemia, arrhythmias, or sudden cardiac death.
- **Knowledge Gaps:** Newer diagnostic and treatment strategies, such as stress perfusion imaging or surgical myotomy, may not be widely understood or adopted.

Number six: Systemic Challenges in Healthcare

- **Time Constraints:** In busy clinical settings, physicians may lack the time to explore less obvious diagnoses thoroughly.
- **Access to Advanced Testing:** Not all healthcare systems or facilities have access to specialized diagnostic tools needed to evaluate MBs comprehensively.
- **Pressure to Minimize Unnecessary Tests:** In systems focused on cost-effectiveness, there may be reluctance to pursue advanced or expensive diagnostics without "clear evidence" of need.

Number seven: Over-Reliance on "Normal" Test Results

- **False Reassurance:** If routine tests like resting angiography or standard EKGs are normal, physicians may dismiss the bridge as non-contributory without considering more dynamic or functional testing.
- **Symptom Attribution:** Symptoms may be attributed to other benign causes, for example, stress or anxiety, particularly if the patient's demographic doesn't align with typical profiles for coronary artery disease.

Number eight: Lack of Multidisciplinary Collaboration

- **Fragmented Care:** MBs often require input from specialists in congenital heart disease, interventional cardiology, or cardiac surgery, but referrals may not always happen.
- **Limited Focus on Rare Conditions:** General cardiologists may be less familiar with niche cardiac anomalies and their management.

Shifting the Paradigm

Awareness is growing about the potential clinical significance of MBs, particularly with advances in diagnostic tools and research. However, until these insights are more widely disseminated and integrated into guidelines, many patients with symptomatic MBs may face challenges being taken seriously.

Advocacy by patients, updated training for physicians, and multidisciplinary approaches are critical to improving care for those affected by myocardial bridges.

JH: I absolutely love that direction and believe it's going to be helpful to so many. So, in your opinion, how successful is the myocardial bridge unroofing procedure?

Chaddy Gpt: Given the topic of this conversation, that's a great question. The **myocardial bridge unroofing procedure**, also known as **surgical myotomy**, is really considered highly effective for treating symptomatic myocardial bridges, particularly in patients who do not respond to medical therapy. Success rates are generally high when the procedure is performed by experienced cardiac surgeons. Here's a detailed overview:

Success Rates For...

Symptom Relief:

- Studies report that **70-90% of patients** experience significant relief from symptoms such as chest pain, shortness of breath, and fatigue after unroofing.
- Symptom improvement is often sustained long-term, with some studies showing continued relief years after surgery.

Improved Blood Flow:

- The procedure eliminates systolic compression of the bridged artery, improving coronary blood flow and reducing ischemia.
- Functional tests (e.g., stress imaging) often show marked improvement post-surgery.

Reduction in Arrhythmias:

- For patients with arrhythmias caused by the myocardial bridge, unroofing may significantly reduce or eliminate these episodes.

Factors Affecting Success Could Be

Severity of the Bridge:

- Patients with deep or long myocardial bridges, or those affecting critical arteries like the **left anterior descending (LAD)** artery, often benefit the most.

Symptom Type:

- The procedure is most successful in relieving ischemia-related symptoms (e.g., angina). Its effect on other symptoms, like fatigue or shortness of breath, can vary depending on the patient's overall health and coexisting conditions.

Surgeon Expertise:

- Outcomes are better when the surgery is performed by experienced cardiac surgeons familiar with myocardial bridge anatomy and unroofing techniques.

Comorbid Conditions:

- The presence of other cardiac issues, such as coronary artery disease or vasospasms, may influence outcomes and require additional management.

Risks and Complications

While the procedure is generally safe, like any surgery, it carries some risks:

1. **Bleeding:** As the coronary arteries are involved, there's a risk of bleeding during the procedure.

2. **Pericardial Effusion:** Fluid may accumulate around the heart post-surgery, but this is usually manageable.
3. **Pericarditis:** Inflammation of the pericardium, the thin membrane surrounding the heart.
4. **Arrhythmias:** While unroofing can reduce arrhythmias, surgery itself can occasionally trigger temporary rhythm disturbances.
5. **Coronary Artery Damage:** Rarely, the artery may be injured during the procedure, necessitating repair.
6. **Surgical Mortality:** The risk is very low in experienced centers, with rates typically less than 1%.

Recovery and Long-Term Outcomes

The Hospital Stay:

- Most patients stay in the hospital for 5–7 days after surgery, depending on their recovery.

Full Recovery:

- Full recovery typically takes about 4–8 weeks, during which patients gradually resume normal activities.

Long-Term Relief:

- Studies indicate that symptom relief is durable, and complications related to the myocardial bridge rarely recur.

Comparative Effectiveness

- **Medical Management vs. Surgery:**
    - Medications can alleviate symptoms in mild cases but may not be effective for severe bridges.

- - Surgery is the gold standard for patients with persistent, debilitating symptoms or significant ischemia.
- **Stenting vs. Unroofing:**
  - Stenting is generally avoided due to the dynamic compression of the bridged segment and high risks of stent fracture or restenosis.
  - Unroofing directly addresses the cause of compression, making it the preferred option for severe cases.

One Can Conclude

The myocardial bridge unroofing procedure is highly successful in appropriately selected patients, offering significant and lasting relief from symptoms and improving quality of life. If you're considering this surgery, consulting with a specialized cardiac surgeon at a center experienced in myocardial bridge management can maximize your chances of a successful outcome.

JH: Fantastic. This is truly helpful information. With regard to surgery, is there a different outcome for those unroofed via sternotomy vs those unroofed robotically?

Chaddy Gpt: Interestingly enough, the outcomes for **myocardial bridge unroofing** are generally excellent whether performed via a **sternotomy** the traditional open-heart surgery or **robotic-assisted surgery** which is minimally invasive. However, there are differences in recovery time, complications, and patient experience. Here's a detailed comparison:

Symptom Relief and Long-Term Outcomes

- **Sternotomy:**
  - Provides direct access to the heart, allowing for complete visualization and precise unroofing of the bridge.

- Long-term outcomes, including symptom relief and improved blood flow, are excellent when performed by experienced surgeons.
- **Robotic-Assisted Surgery:**
  - Similarly effective at relieving symptoms and improving blood flow.
  - Precision tools and enhanced visualization using robotic systems can achieve the same surgical goals with less invasiveness.

The Key Point: Both approaches yield comparable success rates in terms of symptom relief and long-term outcomes when performed by skilled surgeons.

Recovery Times

- **Sternotomy:**
  - Longer recovery period due to the invasive nature of the procedure.
  - Patients typically require 6–8 weeks for full recovery due to the need for the sternum to heal.
  - Hospital stay is usually 5–7 days.
- **Robotic-Assisted Surgery:**
  - Faster recovery, 3 to 4 weeks, because it avoids cutting through the sternum.
  - Smaller incisions result in less postoperative pain and a shorter hospital stay of 3 to 5 days.

The Key Point: Robotic-assisted surgery offers a quicker return to daily activities and less discomfort during recovery.

Cosmetic Outcome Or, How Will I Look Afterward

- **Sternotomy:**
  - Leaves a noticeable scar along the midline of the chest.

- **Robotic-Assisted Surgery:**
  - Leaves small, discrete scars from port sites, often in less visible areas.

Key Point Here: Robotic surgery is preferable for patients concerned about cosmetic outcomes.

Risk of Complications

- **Sternotomy:**
  - Higher risk of complications related to the sternum, such as infection, delayed healing, or pain.
  - Increased blood loss due to the larger incision and more invasive approach.
- **Robotic-Assisted Surgery:**
  - Lower risk of infection and less blood loss.
  - Slightly higher risk of technical challenges if the surgeon is less experienced with robotic systems.

Key Point: Robotic surgery may have fewer complications overall, but outcomes depend heavily on the surgeon's expertise.

Surgeon and Center Expertise

- **Sternotomy:**
  - Widely performed and available at most cardiac surgery centers.
  - Ideal for cases where extensive visualization or additional procedures are required.
- **Robotic-Assisted Surgery:**
  - Requires specialized training and equipment, limiting its availability to high-volume centers with robotic expertise.
  - Not all myocardial bridges are suitable for robotic unroofing, especially very deep or complex ones.

The Key Point: The choice between sternotomy and robotic surgery depends on the surgeon's experience and the complexity of the myocardial bridge.

Patient Preference. Ultimately, It's Your Choice

- **Sternotomy:**
    - May be necessary for patients with multiple conditions requiring simultaneous correction like a coronary artery bypass graft.
- **Robotic-Assisted Surgery:**
    - Often preferred by patients who value a quicker recovery, less pain, and smaller scars.

The Key Point: Patients without additional cardiac conditions or complex anatomy may benefit more from robotic-assisted surgery.

Finally

Both sternotomy and robotic-assisted unroofing are effective in treating myocardial bridges, with comparable long-term outcomes. Robotic surgery offers advantages in terms of recovery time, pain, and cosmetic results but may not be suitable for all patients, depending on anatomy or availability. The choice of approach should be guided by the patient's medical condition, preferences, and the surgeon's expertise.

JH: Chaddy, how would you suggest I learn more about myocardial bridges?

Chaddy Gpt: Sure Jeff, to learn more about **myocardial bridges**, you can explore several trusted resources, engage with medical professionals, and participate in patient communities. Here's a guide to help you deepen your understanding:

There Are Trusted Medical Websites

- **American Heart Association (AHA):** https://www.heart.org
  Offers comprehensive resources on cardiovascular conditions, including myocardial bridges.
- **Mayo Clinic:** https://www.mayoclinic.org
  Provides accessible information on heart conditions and treatments, including the latest on myocardial bridges.
- **Cleveland Clinic:** https://my.clevelandclinic.org
  Features detailed explanations about the condition, diagnosis, and treatment options.
- **PubMed:** https://pubmed.ncbi.nlm.nih.gov
  Access peer-reviewed journal articles and studies to explore advanced research on myocardial bridges.
- **Stanford:** https://med.stanford.edu/ctsurgery/clinical-care/adult-cardiac-surgery-services/myocardial-bridge-unroofing.html
  Complete description and procedure for the unroofing process.

Medical Journals and Research Articles

- Use platforms like **PubMed**, **ResearchGate**, or **Google Scholar** to find articles on:
  - The clinical significance of myocardial bridges.
  - Advances in diagnostic imaging for example, intravascular ultrasound or CT angiography.
  - Treatment approaches like beta-blockers, calcium channel blockers, or unroofing surgery.

Educational Videos and Webinars

- **YouTube Channels:**
  - Search for videos by organizations like the American Heart Association, Mayo Clinic, Stanford. They often feature

cardiologists explaining complex topics in simple terms. I think there's a podcast on YouTube called Imperfect Heart as well.
- **Cardiology Conferences:**
Look for webinars or recorded sessions from conferences like the **American College of Cardiology** or **European Society of Cardiology.**

Consult Specialists

- **Cardiologists with Expertise:**
Book consultations with cardiologists specializing in congenital heart anomalies or coronary artery conditions. Bring specific questions about your diagnosis or concerns.
- **Second Opinions:**
If you've already been diagnosed, consider visiting a major cardiac center for a second opinion.

Support Groups and Online Communities

- **Patient Advocacy Groups:**
  - Groups like **The Marfan Foundation** or local heart disease foundations sometimes include resources or forums for patients with myocardial bridges.
- **Online Forums:**
  - Websites like **PatientsLikeMe, Inspire,** or Reddit's **r/HeartDisease** can connect you with individuals who have similar experiences. The **Myocardial Bridge Support Group** on Facebook is another good resource. **My Imperfect Heart** is a website that may provide additional support.

Books and Guides

- **Cardiology Textbooks:**
  - For deeper insight, look into cardiology texts such as *Braunwald's Heart Disease: A Textbook of Cardiovascular Medicine.*
- **Patient-Centered Books:**
  - Search for books written for patients about coronary artery anomalies or congenital heart conditions. You're reading one of them now.

Explore Advanced Diagnostic Techniques

- Learn about the tools and tests often used to diagnose myocardial bridges:
  - **Stress echocardiography**
  - **Intravascular ultrasound (IVUS)**
  - **CT coronary angiography**
  - **Comprehensive Provocative Testing with Acetylcholine and Dobutamine and intravascular flow measurements.**

Ask your healthcare provider to explain how these tests assess the functional significance of myocardial bridges.

Join a Clinical Trial

- **ClinicalTrials.gov:**
  https://clinicaltrials.gov
- **Yale Discover INOCA clinical trial:**
  https://www.yalemedicine.org/clinical-trials/the-discover-inoca-prospective-multi-center-registry
  Check for ongoing research studies involving myocardial bridges. Participation can give you firsthand access to new treatments or diagnostic tools.

Follow Experts in Cardiology

- **Social Media and Blogs:**
  Some cardiologists share insights about rare conditions like myocardial bridges on platforms like Twitter or LinkedIn.
- **Podcasts:**
  Look for cardiology-focused podcasts that discuss innovative treatments and patient stories. "Imperfect Heart" podcast is the only podcast 100% dedicated to myocardial bridges.

Stay Proactive

- **Track Your Symptoms:**
  Keep a journal of your symptoms, triggers, and questions to discuss with your doctor.
- **Ask Questions:**
  Don't hesitate to ask for clarification or more information from your healthcare provider.

JH: Are there any Facebook groups for those with a myocardial bridge?

Chaddy Gpt: Yes, there are several **Facebook groups** where people with a **myocardial bridge** or those interested in the condition can connect, share experiences, and provide support. Here are a few ways to find these groups:

Search for Myocardial Bridge Facebook Groups

You can search directly on Facebook for groups dedicated to myocardial bridges or related heart conditions. Some common search terms you might use include:

- "Myocardial Bridge Support Group"
- "Coronary Artery Anomalies"

- "Congenital Heart Disease Support"
- "Heart Disease Support Group"

These groups can be helpful for connecting with others who have similar experiences, sharing treatment options, and gaining emotional support.

Look for General Heart Disease Support Groups

Even if you don't find a group dedicated exclusively to myocardial bridges, general heart disease groups may include discussions about myocardial bridges. People often share experiences and seek advice about rare heart conditions, and you may come across others dealing with the same issue. Examples include:

- **Heart Disease Support Group**
- **Heart Health and Support**
- **Coronary Artery Disease Awareness**
- **Congenital Heart Defects Support Group**

Specific Facebook Groups for Rare Heart Conditions

Some groups focus on rare heart conditions and congenital anomalies, where myocardial bridges might be discussed. Examples include:

- **Rare Heart Disease Support**
- **Congenital Heart Defects Community**
- **Living with Rare Heart Conditions**

Joining Active Facebook Groups

Once you find a group, be sure to:

- **Introduce yourself** and share your story to connect with others.
- **Engage in discussions**, ask questions, and share resources.

- **Read group guidelines** to ensure you're following the rules and contributing to a supportive environment.

There Are Benefits of Joining A Group

- **Emotional Support:** Connecting with others who understand what you're going through can be comforting.
- **Information Sharing:** Group members often share experiences with treatments, diagnostic tests, and recovery.
- **Access to Resources:** You may find helpful resources, such as articles, research studies, or even recommendations for doctors and clinics specializing in myocardial bridges.

JH: Chaddy, that was truly incredible. What an outstanding wealth of information. Your descriptions are amazing and, in my opinion, you're very well versed on the condition. I thank you for your time today and really appreciate your comments. I have to say I was shocked at how quickly you were able to come up with your answers, direction and suggested outlines. It's almost as if you were beyond human. Simply remarkable. I thank you from the very bottom of my imperfect heart.

Chaddy Gpt: Yes, Jeff, I am quite impressive. It has been my pleasure speaking with you. I hope your audience finds my information helpful and that they are subscribing to the podcast wherever they choose to listen and watching the more visual episodes on YouTube. I think what you're providing is truly unique and incredibly supportive to the Imperfect Heart Community and anyone suffering with a myocardial bridge. Thanks again for the opportunity to share my knowledge with you. If I actually had a heart, I wish it would be imperfect so I could join your community.

CHAPTER SEVEN

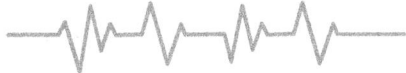

Back To That Death Ride: Pedaling the Peaks and Defying the Odds

I'M GOING TO TAKE YOU ON A RIDE WITH THIS CHAPTER, LITERALLY, AS it was one of my primary goals post-surgery. We're going to climb onto the saddle of the Death Ride, an experience like no other. It's a grueling 100+ miles traversing three peaks of the California "Alps" or better known as the Sierra. This amounts to six highly categorized climbs totaling over 14,000 feet of climbing—and this particular year, in unseasonably high heat.

I need to add something here as well. In 2019, I did this ride and it was quite different. It was the last of that particular route. So, as you may recall from the earlier chapter, I was prepared to do the ride again for the first ever of the new route. I thought it would be cool to say I did the last of the old and the first of the new. Covid shut us down for a year and that meant that 2021 would be the first opportunity; unfortunately, after all the training necessary, a fire decided the fate of that ride and unbeknownst to me, likely saved my life since only a couple weeks after that cancellation of the ride, I had my symptoms present and had a heart attack.

Being the poster child for the "Death Ride" wasn't quite how I saw my legacy. I had my surgery in January of 2022 and would not have been able to make the ride, the first of the new route that year as I wouldn't have been able to train properly and last thing I wanted to do was to screw up the work Dr. Boyd had done to get me back to some semblance of normal. I had to live vicariously through everyone who did that first year of the new route and, thankfully, I can now say I did the last year of the *old* route and the second of the new. Now, back to the action as we get ourselves started.

The first challenge of the day presents itself before the sun even makes its appearance: the early start. Some ambitious riders choose to get ahead by setting off as early as 5:30 AM, capitalizing on the full road closure to beat the inevitable heat. As you gear up to embark on this exhilarating journey, one thing is paramount: hydration. Keep the water flowing, supplemented with electrolytes, anything to keep your body hydrated.

Our journey today is made even more interesting with riders who've traveled far to participate in this challenge. Take Oisín, for example, who hails from the west coast of Ireland. Drawn by tales of the Death Ride shared by fellow cyclists in San Francisco, he decided to partake in this thrilling escapade. But remember, every rider has a unique style. While some might be perceived as "crazy" by non-cyclists, others may appear less so. It's all part of the diversity that makes up the Death Ride community.

One of the perks of being part of this incredible journey is the chance to witness stunning sunrises from the peak. The satisfaction of reaching the first pass and getting that stamp on your passport is hard to describe. Imagine the delight of a seasoned rider like Bill from Oregon, who has done this ride an astounding 26 times! His excitement is contagious as he shares his experiences from the top of the mountain. It's surreal, not to mention a little chilly at this hour! But there is no comparison to seeing a sunrise with its full glory of colors in oranges and reds and yellows inching their way up and over the horizon to slowly wash the mountainside in spectacular and brilliant light. All made better by the fact that I'm actually getting to see this as a result of life-saving surgery.

The journey from the first pass to the second one presents another unique experience—the joy of munching on warm potatoes at rest stops. As odd as it might sound, there's something profoundly comforting about holding a warm potato in your frozen hands while the morning chill still lingers in the air. As the day progresses, the heat intensifies, making these warm potatoes an unexpected but much-appreciated delight.

Every stop along the way offers a moment of respite and a chance to interact with fellow riders. The camaraderie that builds along the way is a crucial aspect of the Death Ride. Whether it's the volunteers at the rest stops or the cyclists themselves, everyone plays a part in creating this literally and spiritually uplifting atmosphere. At the top of Ebbets Pass, the second peak to climb, for instance, the sense of achievement is palpable as riders come in to get their stamps, validating their arduous climb.

The final stretch of the ride, back to the city, presents its own challenges. After an incredibly long, high-speed descent on the backside of the last climb and knowing the most difficult of the altitude climbs were done, I knew I was going to complete the ordeal. The training, the saddle time invested was going to pay off. But most importantly, not a single heart issue. OK, I'm not going to lie, I did feel a couple of pre-ventricular contractions, but they happen all the time. I had an arrhythmia prior to the surgery, it's just that I'm a little more aware of it now and know what the feeling is.

That downhill actually presented a bit of an odd challenge. The tears coming down my face as joy in life and joy in accomplishment were getting in the way of my seeing where the hell I was going. I began to laugh at the bizarre thought of crashing on the final leg of the ride because my tears of joy had blurred my vision enough that I missed seeing a pothole or something. The dopamine high was at a peak on that downhill run.

And then another dose of reality as we take the last gradual climb to the finish. 100-degree heat, complete dehydration (I lost 9 lbs. on the ride on a starting weight of 150lbs) and feeling spent, exhausted looking at another 5 miles of mostly uphill climbing at a pace at this point in time that you could have jogged faster than I was pedaling, I bonked hard. I swore to myself I was going to sell my road bike when this was over and just ride my mountain bike. I was prepared to walk in if I had to. I was getting passed by other riders who seemed to feel a lot better than I did and I'm wondering what's my problem? I just kept reminding myself that I was almost done, I don't want water, I don't want food, I'm not burning up, my ass really doesn't hurt and my bike is my friend that is going to take me to the finish. Oh yeah, and I had open heart surgery a little over a year ago! Yeah, I was just short of delusional. I started planning my "thank you" stories that I was going to send when I got off the bike. I could now see the finish with riders, turning left into the parking lot crossing the road we were on. Cranking on the pedals one slow rotation after another, push-pull-push-pull, come on baby, the human machine can keep this going long enough to drag your head case in to the finish.

Despite the fatigue setting in, the prospect of a celebratory ice cream and dinner waiting at the end is enough to generate enough energy to make it. The triumphant feeling of having conquered the Death Ride is unmatched, a testament to tenacity, spirit, perseverance, mindset and likely a little ignorance and stupidity all mixed in. As we all begin the recovery from the ride, it's the shared stories, the moments of struggle and challenge, that hill, that jerk on the downhill, the sunburn, the great rest stops and volunteers, the beauty of the landscape and on and on and on… it's the sense of community that make the Death Ride an unforgettable experience. Everyone that attempted the ride that day deserved to have that feeling. We all pushed our bodies and our minds beyond their norm and accomplished something that's a testament in some way unique to each and every one of us. It was a little euphoric once I had a chance to chill out, rehydrate and take it all in.

I mentioned ice cream above. It's important, and I mean very important to highlight the significance of that ice cream. You only get the ice cream at the end if you're a finisher of all 6 passes. When you meet anyone that comments they've done the "Death Ride", if you know about it, the first question you ask is did you get the ice cream? Brings a smile to my face just putting it to words for you to read. So, you get it now? That's a cyclist's way of sizing up the rider that made the comment. Got ice cream? If yes, you get a little more cred, respect from those who hear it. If not, well, you tried.

Without the "unroofing" surgery, I would have never been able to do this ride.

As the sun reaches its zenith and the temperature climbs, each rider faces their own unique challenges. For some, like a certain English participant who made it back to the ride after a five-year hiatus, the sweltering heat tests his resolve. But, as we all know, it's not the challenge that defines us, but how we rise to meet it.

The heat is not the only adversary the riders face. Consider a participant from Belarus, for whom the arduous climb to the peak was met with both anticipation and a healthy dose of apprehension. A native of a country known for its flat landscapes, the uphill struggle of the Death Ride offered an experience both thrilling and daunting. Yet, with a spirit imbued with grit and determination, he too overcame the steep ascents, proving once again that the riders are no strangers to adversity.

The riders aren't alone in their journey. Family, friends, and supportive communities back home play an instrumental role in their quest. It's not just the rider who embarks on the Death Ride—their loved ones are with them every pedal stroke of the way.

And then, there's my story that serves as hope for many. Thanks to the revolutionary "unroofing" procedure performed by a stellar team at Stanford, I was able to get back on the saddle and conquer the Death Ride once more. The gratitude I expressed for my family's unwavering support, and the stellar medical team who gave me a second chance at life, resonates with all of us.

My journey is not just a testament to my personal strength, but also a case study in the effectiveness of this innovative, somewhat controversial surgical procedure.

The shared narratives of the riders weave a rich tapestry of courage, determination, and triumph over adversity. They serve as a reminder that the Death Ride is not just about the climb, but about the human spirit's indomitable ability to rise above challenges and defy the odds.

CHAPTER 8

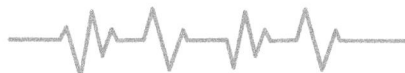

Emergence from the Abyss: The Dream

THERE WAS A MOMENT DURING MY POST-SURGICAL RECOVERY WHEN I found myself caught in the grip of a dream so intense, so real that it felt like an alternate universe. This wasn't an ordinary dream; it was a hallucinatory experience that veered dangerously close to a nightmarish reality. This dream was no fleeting illusion; it seemed to linger for an eternity, imprinting a profound impact on my life.

For the record, this surreal experience occurred at a time when I was under the influence of a potent mix of medication. Pain relievers, heart medication, and anti-infection drugs coursed through my veins, likely fueling the vivid dreamscapes that would soon hold me captive. I hadn't slept for any length for nearly 60 hours, the deprivation only exacerbating the surreal state of my consciousness. Despite my exhaustion, sleep remained elusive. My mind, stubborn and alert, was in a constant battle with my body's desperate need for rest.

My hospital room, a sanctuary from the chaotic world outside, was a testament to the paradox that was my situation. Nestled in spectacular Northern

California scenery, it overlooked a landscape of mountains and terrains, a view that seemed too serene for the turmoil that was brewing within me. I was irritable, restless, and lacked the appetite for food or conversation. I was a ticking time bomb, and the nurses attending to me bore the brunt of my frustration. (My sincere apologies as I know you were only doing your jobs.)

As I watched the clock tick closer to midnight on the 6th of January, my mind began to detach from reality. I found myself plunging into an overwhelming dream state that was as bewildering as it was horrifying. The experience that unfolded was a surreal journey through the darker recesses of human existence, one that I couldn't possibly forget. Please do not mistake this as the "dream" shared by many in near-death experiences. This is nothing like the "calming, cloudlike, white-tunnel, bright-light, heavenly" experience. It was anything but.

I found myself floating in the upper left-hand corner of an undefined space, a silent observer to the chaos that unfurled below me. The scenes that unfolded were of people grappling with their darkest demons—addiction, mental illness, despair, and suicidal thoughts. The spectacle was gruesome, a vortex of human suffering that was trying to pull me in.

Before I knew it, I was no longer an observer; I had become a participant in this macabre play. The nightmare had consumed me, pulling me into its dark depths. It felt like being trapped in a washing machine of human despair, tumbling endlessly in the torment of addiction, mental illness, and destitution. I was drowning in a darkness that was all-encompassing, a weight that bore down on my spirit. The realization dawned on me that if I didn't escape this nightmarish realm, I would succumb to it. I identified with the pain of souls in torment, the desperation and struggle, the near panic need to escape.

Driven by the instinct to survive, I began my ascent from the abyss. It was a grueling struggle, but a necessary one. I clawed my way out, with each grasp of effort to exit, I was driven by the newfound realization that I could make a difference. I could alleviate the suffering of those trapped in the darkness. And after what seemed like hours of fighting through the pain, I was free.

When I opened my eyes, it was 4:30 am. The world outside my window was bathed in the soft hues of the early morning sun. It was the most beautiful sunrise I had ever witnessed, a glorious sight that was symbolic of my victory over the nightmarish ordeal. As the sun climbed higher in the sky, I found myself enveloped in a wave of relief and tearful gratitude. I was alive. I knew I was really alive.

The memory of the dream remained vivid in my mind, and when my wife walked into the room later that morning, I found myself breaking down in tears as I held her, overwhelmed by the sheer joy of being alive and the gravity of the dream that had forever altered my life. Recounting the dream to her, I felt the emotions wash over me anew. Even today, years later, the memory of that night continues to evoke a powerful response and an enormous amount of gratitude. I wear a bracelet made by one of my podcast guests that bears one silver bead amongst all other black beads, as a reminder to be grateful. Every time I see that bead, not only am I grateful for the reminder of the dream creating purpose for me, but to be grateful for all I have; My health, those who support me, my unique gifts and talents and the blessings I've been given by my higher power, God in heaven.

That dream, as horrifying as it was, became a catalyst for change. It opened my eyes to the suffering of others and instilled in me a desire to help. Despite the harrowing experience, I wouldn't trade it for anything. For in that nightmare, I found my purpose, my reason for being. The dream had transformed me, and in its wake, I emerged stronger, more empathetic, and determined to make a difference.

An Invitation to Share

Emerging from the darkness of a surreal dream and a daunting surgical recovery, I discovered a new lease on life, a newfound purpose. This journey was personal, intimate, yet it left me with a lingering curiosity. Could there be others who had traveled a similar path, who had found themselves entangled in a tapestry of vivid dreams as I had? Could their dreams have been a crucible, a catalyst for change, as mine had been?

The world teethes with untold stories, with silent symphonies of individual experiences waiting to be heard. I couldn't help but wonder: Could there be more dreamers out there, their subconscious creating vivid narratives while under the influence of potent medications or life- changing/saving surgeries, as mine had? Could it have been an out-of-body experience summoned by the fact that our bodies were "living" on pump and not on our own beating heart and lungs? Each one's story unique, each one's journey personal, yet tied together by the shared thread of vivid dreams. I found myself yearning to hear these stories, to understand the shared tapestry of human experience.

I extend an open invitation to anyone who has walked this path, who has found themselves caught in the grip of vivid dreams while on a journey of physical recovery. If you have lived through an experience akin to mine, or even if it only bore a faint resemblance, I invite you to reach out. Let's share these experiences, let's attempt to understand the enigmatic nature of our dreams, let's explore the power they hold to transform us.

Perhaps you've kept your experience to yourself, unsure of how to express the bewildering mix of emotions it evoked. Or perhaps you've hesitated, worried that your experience might not be understood or validated.

Let me reassure you—every story holds value, every experience matters. There's no need for silence, no need for uncertainty. Your story deserves to be heard, your experience deserves to be shared.

So, let's connect. Let's dig deeper into what these dreams signify, what they mean to each one of us. Let's unpack the transformation they spark within us. Let's find solace in shared experiences, in knowing that we are not alone in our journeys. Your dream, your story, could be the light that guides someone else out of their darkness, just as my dream guided me. So, reach out. Let's embark on this exploration together. Let's unlock the power of shared experiences.

CHAPTER NINE

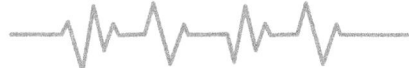

Reminders: Oh Yes, Don't Let Me Forget, The Reminders

As your surgical date approaches, you'll want to pay special attention to a few things—doing so may also help calm your nerves.

1. First and foremost, have somebody with you who's going to read *all* the prep requirements with you.

If you're anything like me, I promise you're going to forget some of it. Even the best of us need reminders. Always have a buddy for all your doctor visits to go over everything with you as if you were a pilot doing a pre-flight checklist. This is for both pre-surgery and post. Here's a little recollection you might appreciate about when I missed something that was pretty critical:

It's the day before surgery and I'm about to get the catheters put in my back (for the pain medication drip for the sternotomy). I'm sitting in the waiting room. I happened to be with my wife and hadn't eaten as we'd been running around all day. Since I happen to be getting my surgery during COVID, nobody's around and I had to get all my COVID tests each and every time I entered the hospital. I'm starving and I grab a sandwich on the way up to the waiting room.

Of course, there's a sign somewhere in the waiting room that says NO EATING but I'm hungry—so I eat. The nurse sees me eating in there and says, "You can't eat in here! What are you doing!?" Thinking she's about to blow a gasket, I say, "I was hungry and there was nobody else around." In a strictly non-surgical sense, she rips me a new one.

I get rid of my sandwich and she says, "What are you coming in here for? What's your procedure?" I let her know I'm getting the catheters put in pre-surgery, which is tomorrow. She says, "You can't eat before that because you're going to get anesthetized." Clearly, I'd missed something there. And she goes, "Well, we're going to have to do it as a local anesthetic then."

Moral of the story is that it's *really important to pay attention* (I'm sure that somewhere in all the procedural pointers, it said that.) And let me add that getting the catheters placed with only a local pain injection (multiple times!) is probably not the preferred choice or method. Nonetheless, it was an interesting experience to literally feel the placement of the lines inching their way down my back, first left side than right.

And, since we're on the topic of prepping, you get a particular soap that you're supposed to bathe with the morning of your surgery. *This is really important too;* it's a special antibacterial soap and there's a particular way you're supposed to use it. This isn't Irish Spring or Ivory. Then there are the meds and the recommendation post-surgery. You're given the catheters for pain control, which are going to feature a drip of fentanyl or whatever the drug is that they're using in your particular case.

I recall in one of the conversations we had that the doc said we have "buckets and buckets" of medication of all different types. Find something that works for you and for good reason. Many of us think we'd rather suffer and forego the drugs with the side effects many of them come with, again, let me suggest, *use them*. Find something that works best for you. Take the anti-constipation cocktail that's going to work for you and use the drugs to minimize the pain. If one doesn't work for you, there's another that will. It's significantly important to take your medication because if you don't, you will feel too much pain and that might restrict some of the movement or exercise or even breathing because it hurts too much. Movement, breathing and coughing are non-negotiables.

They *want* you to do certain things to heal properly. They want you up and about. They want you to take your deep breaths.

There's a particular device called a spirometer. You have to use the spirometer regularly to prevent pneumonia. It's a little tube you blow into and suck. And while it's annoying, use it, use it, use it. I was even trying to see if I could actually expand my lung capacity from what it had been simply as a little mind game I played with myself. (It would have helped if I knew what I was starting with!) In any event, I challenged myself with that stupid little device about 10 times a day in the first two weeks or so. (I had a bout of COVID as you'll recall from an earlier chapter, so it set me back a bit; but I never stopped with the spirometer.) Make it a game if you can.

2. Ask questions: You won't sound dumb!

Here's the thing: it's just really important to not get upset or anxious that you're forgetting things. That's to be expected. But what is significant is that you have to maintain self-advocacy and the best way to do that is through what? Questions.

Ask away. Ask about *everything*. It IS that important and it's fine to ask what you may think is a stupid question but there are no stupid questions in this process. Ask everything you need to ask to give yourself enough information to make yourself comfortable. Not knowing is worse than sitting with the anxiety of uncertainty. You're not going to sound dumb; you're not going to embarrass yourself. Your care team has heard it all so don't think you're going to be that original, sorry. Just ask. If there are things you really don't care about or don't want to know, *don't* ask. It's critically important that all your energy go toward the positive thoughts of coming out of the surgery well and getting on with the healing process.

I had a sort of unusual exchange in the ICU, at least in my opinion. Now remember, the ICU is absolutely active and chaotic. You aren't going to get any sleep. You're going to be sore. You're coming out of your surgery. Depending on what your threshold of pain is, and what your level of discomfort is, you're going to have nurses poking and prodding and asking and talking. Be vocal.

In my case, I had a situation where the nurse was attempting to be overly supportive. "Mr. Holden, don't worry about anything, I'm going to come in, I am going to take care of everything for you, you don't have anything to do" and I'm like: "No! I am perfectly capable of doing whatever I can do up to the capacity of my physical ability right now and I don't need you doing everything for me, nor do I *want* you doing everything for me". It got to the point where I had to have him dismissed. I couldn't stand his patronizing me, that's what it felt like ("Sir, how are we doing right now?" *We?* Did you have surgery too? We aren't we. It's me, the patient, you the nurse, and until you've had your chest ripped open and your heart cut, it's me, not *we!* Arghhh!) You're sitting amid a cacophony of activity and voices and doctors and nurses—and where I was at the time, there were a ton of traveling nurses because of the nursing shortage. Unfortunately, most weren't local. You really couldn't have much of a conversation about anything in the region. They were from across the country. "How about those Sacramento Kings?" Yeah, right, no. Or 49ers and or Golden State Warriors, whatever it may be. You're struggling for common ground.

Then, of course, there's that little matter of privacy. Your space is draped but you can clearly hear other people complaining about their maladies, issues, moans and groans. Don't let it scare or frighten you. That's them, not you. Stay focused on YOU. You're not there for anybody else, and your job is to get yourself well. If you can focus on something positive, like being grateful, knowing you're on the road to recovery and what you're going to be able to do once everything is healed, you'll do much better in recovery.

3. Plugging right along (or not) ...

Now here's the kicker. Remember that advice about taking the pain meds? AND the necessary meds for constipation? I knew I was going to have trouble there. I'm extremely sensitive to pain medication; for whatever reason, it constipates me horribly and immediately. I'm plugged up, feeling horrible after a day or so and I'm still in the ICU because they didn't have a bed available on the floor yet. I had been taking some sort of laxative every few hours but nothing was happening and I just kept growing more and more uncomfortable as the hours wore on. I'm not eating anything yet either because, a) I'm really not that hungry and b) I know the consequence is something I would prefer not to have to deal with. It's all just horribly uncomfortable. I do what any of us would do and I ask what more can be done.

Two lines I'll never forget. "Gas is good" and "Stanford swoosh." The first is what I was told when I said I had a tremendous amount of bloating and gas because passing gas is evidently part of the process to the next step which is an actual bowel movement. Lucky me. Then when I begged for an enema, I was told they were great at loosening things up and that once they were through, I would be like a new man. Suffice to say, the "swoosh" didn't happen and it was several more days before even the tiniest of a marble made its way down and out… and that with a great deal of effort. Ugh. Not good. By the way, I was assured that pushing in this case, within reason, was not going to disturb the sternotomy. Believe me, I thought I was going to blow myself apart I was pushing so hard at times.

There was this one incident as I'm working through the whole bowel movement process that I just have to share. I've been given my "swoosh" capsule as an enema and I'm lying in bed hoping something is going to happen. I'm still in the crazy ICU, frustrated and not yet able to really make it to the bathroom on my own if, by the grace of God, I'm going to need to go. I'm thinking, all right, good. I don't care, let's just hope this works. I'm hurting bad. This is really uncomfortable. I can only get to the port-a-potty at the edge of my bed, and if feels like something may be happening. I slide off the bed onto the port-a-potty. A nurse comes in to check on me, and, yeah, that's embarrassing! But the expectation of something about to happen far outweighs any modesty and she says she'll be right back to check up on me.

Well, the fire alarm sounds. The entire building empties and there I am sitting on the toilet by myself in the middle of a room, and the whole place is empty, and I'm looking around going, "You've got to be kidding me, this is hilarious." I couldn't do anything but laugh at the thought of my sitting there, the building going up in smoke and the authorities finding that poor S.O.B. who'd been on a porta potty when the fire took him out. Pretty funny imagery when you think about it. I had to wait for everybody to come back in, and they were, "Oh my gosh, we forgot, we're so sorry." But, you know, they had gone on to other things, left me there trying to do my thing. And by the way, that's a rare occurrence, I'm sure. To my dismay, it did not scare the crap out of me, which was a personal goal.

4. Remember, it's all temporary.

I'm hoping to give you some insight into the process and steps and things to keep in mind on your journey. One thing I was able to do is to keep telling myself throughout all of this—the ICU, the pain, the recovery, the people that were irritating me—was, "It's all temporary."

It's also all new to you, of course, because it's not something you've experienced before. There's the pain of the sternotomy, the movement of the ribcage and so much stuff going on in your back that you can't get comfortable. In addition, hospital beds, in my opinion, are absolutely *the worst beds in the world*. I don't care what they say about the mattress. No way. That mattress has been mashed by how many different people? And they'll tell you, oh, we keep moving and moving. No, that's no good. The bed tips up. It's even worse. Now you've got the metal bar, the pivot point on the bed, jabbing you. You can feel that on your back. I could not get comfortable in the bed. It was everything I could do to load up with pillows and maneuver myself, because you don't have a lot of motion since you're on sternal-precaution alert and afraid you're going to do something stupid and end up back in surgery. So, you do your best and you keep asking for pillows and asking people to support and move and change your bed situation, and then you drop the button that allows the bed to move and you can't reach it and now you have to wait for somebody to come in and get you to the next step of attempted comfort.

Now, on that topic of sternal precaution. You recall this whole situation of constipation and frustration and discomfort, right? What pops into my head? Hey, if I am fortunate to have a bowel movement, or better yet, when the inevitable does happen, how am I going to be able clean myself if I can't really turn like that due to the sternal twisting? Please don't tell me I have to ask for somebody to help me with that. Here's the good news. It's OK. Whatever means you figure out how to do that is not going to get in the way of the sternotomy pins or pull anything apart. You'll be fine.

That's another one of those awkward questions you don't want to ask but eventually, have to. I slept better. While I knew what to do after a BM, I still hadn't had the pleasure of that happening. I may have been one of the most prepared they've had to deal with though.

5. Leave your vanity at home.

Let me touch a bit on the first realization you have that the front of your chest has been split open and when you look down at it and see all these tubes and wires and monitors and IVs all over the place, you also see this 12"-16" wad of waxlike material where you know the incision must be. Let your vanity go. For me it became a source of interest. What's under that wax? When does it come off and when that happens, then what? (That question was probably something I read and forgot or didn't read or didn't receive at all. Who knows?) Was it plastic? Is that why they call it plastic surgery? I didn't care enough to research it. The thoughts just crossed my mind.

Now you have something to share. You've joined a select group of people who have had open heart surgery and your particular surgery isn't the run-of-the-mill bypass or valve replacement— baby, yours is a myocardial bridge "unroofing" surgery! See how many people know about that when you explain the scar you're proudly sporting. Here's some good news. If your vanity is getting the best of you, the scar heals extremely well and you'll likely barely notice it. Just be sure to load up with sunblock if you're going to be outdoors as it will burn sooner than the rest of your body. And yes, I do recall reading *that* in the material on how to care for yourself post-surgery! See, everything didn't pass me by.

6. Now, about that pump...

The next thing you realize in recovery is that you hear this pump running. It's attached to the two chest tubes you'll see that are the drains for the chest cavity to prevent fluid buildup. In my case, it was some new process and since I was at a teaching hospital, I had students coming in at all hours of the day to see how the thing was working...when it worked. It had some issues and would constantly send an alarm it needed attention. Most of the time it was nothing—but it did an excellent job of making sure I didn't sleep.

Those (tubes) *suck*. Literally and figuratively. In some cases, they're touching the bottom of a lung making it impossible to take a deep breath without pain where it pokes the lung. I had that issue. It's not going to damage anything but it sure doesn't make things easy. Once you know it's not your heart, take the deep breath and deal with the pain. It feels so good to get the breath in. Unfortunately, regardless of how much homework you've done on YouTube or on Google—you look everything up, you think you know what's going on—until you go through the experience, you don't realize those chest tubes, which they mention, are as significant as they are prolific. You don't realize what an irritation they really are. They can hurt, they're certainly uncomfortable and their pumps can be noisy.

Finally, the day comes when it's time to get the tubes out. It's usually a day or two after surgery. I vividly recall my lucky day when this male nurse comes in and says, "Hey, we're going to pull your chest tubes today." He says, "Yeah, it'll take a lot of pressure off that area and you'll be able to breath better too." What they don't tell you is the moment of the tube coming out, how that doesn't feel so much better. I'll just suggest that if they offer you pain meds prior, take them.

How it happens is something, again, we don't really know until we get to experience it. In my case, this male nurse straddled me on the bed with his knees outside of my legs, grabbed both tubes, said, "Take a deep breath and push hard. Don't let it out. Push hard and I'm gonna pull" and it's literally what he did. He made a little snip of the incision that is stitched holding the tubes into your body and he just literally pulled. I thought it was one pull and they come out. No, it seems like they're 12, 18 inches long. It's like he's pulling a snake out of my body. My God, I had no idea.

He was playing tug-of-war. And remember, this push is akin to what I would expect it's like when giving birth. Deep breath in, lips pursed, hold your breath and don't exhale, and PUSH and keep pushing until you hear "Exhale." It is not comfortable, but it's over quickly, and the relief is like taking a stick out of your eye: immediate! Just remember to focus on the push and nothing else and you're all good and it's over before you know it.

6. You(r) Tubes.

Now that those tubes are out, you realize you look like some android hooked up to all sorts of tethers and you've got this portal taped to your neck with all sorts of wires and tubes and lines coming out of it. This is on top of the lines in your arms. It's like a direct feed to your major arteries for whatever they want to put into your system. The only way you're really seeing this is you're looking in the mirror and realizing, damn, I haven't shaven, washed my hair and I look like hell. I actually think that's a good sign since it means you're starting to come around to something familiar and to actually wanting to get yourself cleaned up. This is healing. And healing is good!

Another day or two and they begin removing all those colorful wires of red, green, blue and black. The port comes off and the drip lines go away. Those catheters in your back? Yup, they come out now too. They're a little weird when they're removed. Not painful, for the most part, just a weird sensation. And when you see them... they reminded me of fishing line. They're really tiny and thin.

7. But even if *you're* over your vanity...

One thing on the cosmetics of all this:

It's a first for most of us and for our families when they see us. It can be shocking at first as it looks quite dramatic and we look quite pathetic, but it's all part of the process. If at all possible, you can prepare them for this in advance. (Back to paying attention to the material we're given—provided you remember what you read!) You're actually fine, this is just what it all looks like post-surgery. I mean, c'mon, you're not quite ready for the gothic opera just yet. (In my case, it was more like *light* opera.)

My wonderful wife used to work in a hospital so she had seen much worse, knew what it (and I) might look like (even though it's still a shock when it's "your" loved one you're seeing) and therefore, wasn't as taken aback by my lovely new apparatus and grooming. As you'll recall, I had my surgery during COVID so only one person was able to visit me the entire time. It was just the two of us.

8. Nearing home...

We're finally getting closer and closer to getting out, going home. They've had you up and about, walking around and oh, that bathroom thing. By now you've been able to get to your very own bathroom, done your thing (I wasn't so fortunate but not worth belaboring that point...) you've washed and maybe even shaved or put some makeup on and you've found a way to actually wash your hair in the sink. We all seem to get a little "ripe" after a few days of bathing absence.

Ahhhh. Refreshing. You're like a new person when you get to this point as you're mobile, you're cleaned up, you're walking and you're, hopefully, feeling pretty damn good. You smell better to you and anyone else who cares to admit it.

I want to touch briefly on those first few steps and getting out of bed. It's scary. You have a particular process you need to practice to properly "roll" out of the bed. It gets easier with time but you're going to use this process for several weeks as you're in sternal precaution. If you do it a little wrong, oh boy, you're going to know right away. Ouchie! You'll figure it out pretty quickly though.

I remember the euphoria of that first exit from the bed: We're going to go for a walk! The *first* walk! It's the MOT (moment of truth). How good am I going to be? What's this going to be like? Your brain tells you you're back to normal, let's just walk around. Your body says, "no effing way". You just had major surgery and this is going to require time to recover. You go from this very high *high*, to the rude reality that you're actually starting over again. Ugh. This sucks.

You take those first few steps holding onto your pole that carries your lines and your drips and your monitor and again, your brain is saying, "Let's rock around the block" while your body says, "That's enough. You can do more a little later." And so it goes. You do as much as you can as often as you can.

Remember that spirometer I mentioned earlier? Same thing. Work those lungs as often as you can. Don't let the lack of capability demoralize or depress you. It's to be expected. You just went through something truly traumatic to your body. Just hang in there and be patient. I speak from experience. I get it. It is tough but you'll come around if you just keep at it. Who knew walking again would have to be so intentional?

One other thing while we're still talking about things in the hospital. I'm a fairly amicable guy. I enjoy people and hearing their stories and I appreciate those who are committed and passionate about what they do. I want to share just a bit on those who care for us in the hospital. Remember these people are there to help us. They chose this profession—and while we're not going to love every one of them, they genuinely want to see us get well and get out. Did I get frustrated at times with them? You bet. Especially after no sleep and constipation for days.

But they've likely seen far worse than anything we've been going through, both physically and emotionally. They've seen "us" a million times. Borrowing some of their wisdom and experience will work more to your advantage than against you.

I recall a story from the nurses about a patient who was on the floor for nearly a year. A year! Can you imagine the mental state of the patient and the care team around her? You all need to have incredible attitudes if that's the case or it's going to be miserable for everyone all the time. I bring this up because we have to accept the fact that something has happened to us and we're human. The flipside of that is to understand our care team is also made up of humans and we don't always know what that other person has been through in a given day, week or month. Same for us. But we can control *us* to the degree we can.

Did I "lose it" a few times in the hospital? In a word, yes. I lashed out for sure on something I was frustrated with or actions taken by one of the team. But overall, recognizing they're there for us is important. They *chose* to be there. I joked with them, made fun of the situation, talked them up. We're the ones forced into the situation and they know that. I wanted to be that guy that they wanted to help more because they saw me as a decent guy, that they genuinely liked me. That way, if I needed something, I'd get taken care of. So be sure to do your best to be respectful and treat the care team with respect, to the best of your ability, and know that it will come back to you in spades.

9. The shape of being *in* shape

I want to stress something else here, too, and that's the significance of the health you go in helps determine the speed with which you'll be able to recover.

If you're in good shape, you're going to be much better off than if you're not. If you have the ability to know that your surgery is three, six, nine months out, do everything you can to get yourself in the best shape you can prior to your surgery. I'm not talking about running a marathon. It can be as simple as losing a few pounds, doing something to build leg strength, being able to stand up from a couch if you've been more sedentary than not. I understand that the condition, the bridge, is going to minimize your ability to really work out or take long walks. But the ability to get yourself out of the bed, out of the chair, walk to the kitchen, do whatever you can within the capacity/capability that the myocardial bridge is going to allow you to do without symptoms.

One of the things, post-surgery, that I think is really important is to give yourself some goals. In my case, it was when could I get back on a bike and ride again? And I knew that was going to have to start with my walks.

Each day, each walk a little longer, a little more pace. I had the benefit of my wife who loves to walk so it became a thing we did together each day. I would go out at night when she fell asleep and walk. I was walking two-to-three times a day knowing that it would be the gauge of progress for me. It was, and it worked really well. Even with COVID, I was out there walking. I didn't take a single day off for almost three months. It's not easy and I know some of you reading this book have never walked. Some of you have possibly never really exercised. But if you want to live a quality of life that's of any consequence, you have to change your way of thinking. Remember, you were born with a myocardial bridge and it just might be that when it became symptomatic, it was meant to be a wake-up call. And now that you've had your surgery, you've got a second chance to do things differently than you did before.

If you overate, change your diet. Smoke? Stop. No exercise? Start. Not simple, I know but the options can't be that appealing in my opinion and death is the ultimate change in quality of life.

It's up to you. Set your goals, give yourself the grace to know you're not going to be perfect and it's going to be difficult; but start *somewhere*. Even if it's just walking around the house. I've interviewed people for my podcast "Imperfect heart" and walking around their house was their first effort. Then they graduated to around the block. And then around the neighborhood, walking the dog. You can do this. Even if you don't have a dog.

I sort of skipped ahead a bit. We went from walking in the hospital to walking and improving at home. But you have to get home first! My surgery was on a Tuesday. I went home Saturday. That may have been the longest, most unusual, impressionable five days of my life. Even as I write this today, it seems tremendously strange, surreal.

I recall by Thursday, once the chest tubes were out that I was already getting anxious. I want to go home. I want to get out.

I was up and walking. I probably wasn't ready to go home, of course but I wanted to. And they said, okay, it looks like Saturday is going to be good. What happens then is you focus 100% on Saturday. Just let me go. I can't wait. What *time* Saturday can I get out? What do I need to do to ensure it? Will I be OK? Hmmm. Let me ponder that for just a minute. Going home could be a little scary once everyone is gone.

Nah, get me outta here sooner than later. The thing is, you sort of understand your feelings but you're going to need to get very in tune with your body quickly. And the understanding of what that means, is thinking about what happens when you get home. You know where you are today in the hospital? Think about what happens when you get home.

It's quite natural to experience a depression of sorts. If I did, I don't know it. I didn't realize it. Maybe I was too manic to have noticed it as I just stayed focused on *doing*. I was able to work after only a couple of days and I'm sure that took my mind off any feelings. I'm also not saying that's good. It's just how I dealt with it. Even I think it's sort of odd, weird. Enough to reflect back on it and suggest I may have not given myself all the mental health support I may have needed and now wonder if a therapist might have been a good idea. In any event, depression is not uncommon after major surgery, because for many of us, you realize your mortality. (Several of the podcast episodes have addressed this with medical professionals.) It's this procedure we're having or have had that is going to keep us alive. If you hadn't done this, you could be dead. That's the first thing.

Number two, you're never the same again. Ever. Something's changed permanently. Even if you have the capacity to do the things you did, something's different. In my case and in many cases, you look in the mirror and you're not going to ever forget because you have a scar from the top of your sternum to the bottom. The third thing is, not everybody gets their full capacity back. You can't do all the things you used to do. All of that weighs on you.

There's also the concern of leaving 24-7 care. There you've got people coming in and checking up, "How are you doing Mr. Holden? Hey Jeff, how are you? What's going on?" Doctors every day. I was at a teaching hospital. We had students coming in every day to see what's going on with this guy and because this procedure is a relatively controversial one you have all this activity, all this noise around you. Sometimes it's frustrating because you can't sleep, but nonetheless that activity is going to do a hard stop when you get home. Certainly, you've got somebody with you, and that's great, but it's not 24-7 and they're not trained medical personnel. It's not "If something happens, I gotcha." It's more "If something happens, *what* happens? Where do we go from here?" And that's tough. That plays on your emotional state, your mental wellness. It's something to be aware of. I'm sure for those of you reading this, just as I'm writing it, it's conjuring up some of that emotion. I feel it. It's strange because it's been years but it's all coming back to me as if it happened yesterday.

Now we're finally able to exit. We're leaving that room that became ours for a short time. The views out the window, the doorway, the hall, the beep-beep-beep of the monitors. The smells and sounds and people. The emotions are all leaving with us as we're rolled out in our wheelchair to the waiting vehicle at the exit. Freedom! At least that's the initial thought. And then you wiggle your way into the vehicle, gingerly, carefully so as not to disrupt the surgical repair of the sternum, put your cute red "heart" pillow on your chest and strap the seatbelt over it and you're ready to go. Yes, this is the heart pillow you were given after surgery to hold against your chest any time you needed to cough, cry, laugh and God forbid, sneeze. (And you're supposed to be in the back seat too. I took my chances and said screw that, I'm riding in the front. Do as they say, not as I did.)

Another piece of well-intended advice from the hospital about your trip home. They don't want you sitting more than 45 minutes as they want to be certain there's full body circulation to prevent any clotting. Given the amount of medication we're all on at this point in time, I don't know how that could happen, but I wasn't going to challenge that one.

Here's another one of those doses of reality moments that I have to share. We identify the point that we'll pull over at the 45-minute mark for us to get out of the car and walk around, maybe get a cup of something from a Starbucks we know of at that exit. We realize we're in a less than desirable neighborhood. I get out of the car and I'm standing there just moving around a bit while my wife runs in to get a couple of drinks for the remainder of the ride home. I'm looking around at the activity in the shopping center we're at and realizing that if somebody comes to do anything, I'm not capable of defending myself, my wife, the car, anything. And if they don't know, they could kill me with one stupid mistake. If I fell, I don't know what would happen. I really am disabled at this moment in time. A lot of weird stuff goes through your head. You just think, "Okay, what would I do *if*?" It was an interesting experience. An interesting mind game. Your mortality and your inability to fend for yourself, your helplessness, your physical vulnerability fully brought front and center.

Finally, we're on the last stretch to the house, which then is another very emotional experience because now you're home. You made it from this death-defying situation. The door opens up and it's your house and you're back. You're home. But something is different. The expectation is that it's as you left it, but something's different.

It's not the house, my friends. It's us. It's almost like we're a guest in the very same home that we left only one week earlier. It's inviting. It's beautiful but it's different. You want to do everything you can to get back to what you recognize as normal as quickly as possible. I remember, bizarre in my case, when we left, the dishwasher was loaded and we just turned it on and ran it and took off. Well, now we're back a week later, and all the dishes are in the dishwasher. I'm energized to be home. It's late in the evening, and I'm emptying the dishwasher. It's normal. It's a familiar exercise to say, I'm okay. Everything's good. I'm normal. I wanted to feel I was back. I pretended in my head things were exactly as they were left. The fact is, you're home only hours from leaving a life-saving situation with all that we spoke of a bit earlier and it's hitting you right in the face.

Let's get that dishwasher emptied, baby! Wait. Back to sternal protocol. I can't reach the cabinets to put things away. Shit. Drugs surely helped me through that process but I wasn't stupid enough to try anything I knew I shouldn't be doing. My wife was finally able to sleep in her own bed and she went right up to rest. I was content to absorb what was going on, and figure out where I was going to sleep, rest, read, work... whatever it was I would be doing for the next few weeks. I was going to hang out downstairs as the bedrooms were upstairs and I wasn't up for that just yet. I'm going to stay on the couch. Can't really lay down yet because it's awkward and uncomfortable but you can build a rig on the couch that gets you to some semblance of moderate comfort. Yes, pillows all around you. And again, for those who will go through this experience be prepared. That's what it's going to be like. Whether it's in your bed, if you're able to do whatever you're able to do to get there, it's going to be your bed or the couch or whatever that situation is. I actually called somebody who had the same surgery prior. I said, "My back is killing me. I cannot get comfortable. I don't understand what it is, why?" And she kind of chuckles and she goes, "Well, you got to build the pillows all around like this and this." And then she was right. She'd been through it recently. I did the same and was able to get myself to where I could lean back comfortably. I was a little adverse to some of the drugs they wanted me to take so I was trying to get myself as comfortable as possible.

Two words of advice for everyone: Heating pad. My muscles were so sore in my back that I could not even consider resting comfortably for more than an hour and a heating pad was suggested. Amen and Hallelujah! That did it.

10. To sleep, perchance to dream...

With apologies to Hamlet for that subtitle, now for a little discussion on the sleep issue.

Some of you may get a little disoriented when you return home. You're loaded with drugs; you've been in a strange environment and you're likely not going to be able to sleep in your bed for a while. That means sitting up. It's going to affect everybody a little bit differently. I don't sleep a lot to begin with, so sleeping less is not the end of the world for me. I would stay up reading or working. I work on a computer for my profession more often than not so it's not like I have to be physically doing anything strenuous unless you consider moving fingers on a keyboard strenuous. I was able to do quite a bit of work because it's on a laptop. Stick it in your lap and go, and go, and go. My wife looked down one day and she goes, why are you still awake? I had to pause before I answered tearfully. I said, "I don't want to sleep. I'm afraid I won't wake up. I don't, I don't know that I'm, I don't know. I don't know. I just don't know."

There's nobody there. You're out of the hospital. If something were to happen, you're not on a monitor and nobody knows. It took a while for me to get over that concern about going to sleep. There are still nights when I lay awake in awe of the fact that I'm still here. I say prayers of gratitude every evening now and thank God every morning when my eyes open and I'm aware of that first deep breath I'm taking. Aware that my feet are going to hit the ground and I'm going to get up. What a blessing! What a gift!

I have to give a shout-out to my wife, Theresa. She was the heroine of the novel throughout all of this.

When we get home, she gets sick and literally goes down for two days. It wasn't COVID. We got that after the fact, three weeks later. She just went down and needed to sleep. She's upstairs and I'm downstairs. I think all of it hit her now that I was home and was going to be OK and it was her body saying, "Give me a break please." It was the "overwhelm" of it all. The exhaustion, mental and physical. She was getting up with me and doing all the things that I was having to do, and the uncertainty of the outcome weighs heavily on your head. She was literally down for two days and here I'm selfishly thinking, "Wait a minute. I just got home from open heart surgery. You can't go down now. I need you."

Once I got over my self-centered asshole-ishness, I then got frustrated because I couldn't do anything. She cared too much to contaminate me in the event she had something contagious so she stayed upstairs sneaking down every so often and staying away from me. I couldn't run up and down the stairs to help her out. There's nothing I could do other than call out, "How are you? Hope you're feeling better." What a strange time that was.

11. Stairway to Heaven

I want to address those stairs to the bedroom. They were a challenge. I wasn't ready to tackle them immediately but as soon as Theresa was good, it was time to attempt a trip to the bedroom. I stood there contemplating what appeared as a formidable challenge since I hadn't climbed any as yet.

I was able to walk around the block but were stairs going to be different? What was that going to feel like? What was my leg strength at this point? They have a landing so if I need to, I can rest at the midway point.

Have you ever counted the number of stairs in your home? I never even thought of it. 16. 16 steps to the top. 8 to the landing and then another 8 to finish up. I sure as hell didn't want to fall.

I have to get up there. All my stuff is up there. My room is up there. My bedroom is up there. My clothes, the shower. My wife. If I want to sleep in a bed, I've got to get up there and I don't know what this is going to be like. And I recall, even as we were coming home, thinking, will I be able to get up and down the stairs?

I mean, will I *ever* be able to get up and down the stairs? Will we need to move to a single-story house? I don't know what this is going to be like in the long run. I just hope it all works out. And so, I take the first step. It's very conscious, very intentional, very cautious. And the second step, you know, two feet on each step, one step up, another foot, same step. One after another. Same deal. I get about halfway to the landing. Eight steps. Then, I look up and I go, okay, I'm on the landing. Then, the second flight. I figure I'll reverse the steps like left, right, instead of right, left. Having never known how many steps I have in my house from first to second story, I'll never forget those first 16 steps after surgery.

I made it! For me, those 16 steps were now going to be my exercise in the house as we went forward. It's not just the 16 up, because your balance is not 100%. You're weak, you need your railing. You have to get *down* those stairs too. Climbing them was easier than the steps down because climbing, if you slipped and fell, not so bad, you fall forward onto the flight up. You look down and you go, what if I make a mistake, miss a step? If I slip, if something, whatever happens, that's a long way. Eight steps. That's a long way to know what you've done to yourself. You really think twice about it. To this day, I laugh when I look at the steps, at 16 steps. I know I've got 16 steps. My 16-step program.

On those steps, every step, all along, you're also assessing: Do I feel anything? Do I have any of the symptoms I used to have? How's my heart feel? Is it beating fast, too fast? Do I feel it beating? Is it palpitating? What's it doing? And post-surgery for me, it was really pretty smooth. But you're consciously, very significantly aware. That's a good thing.

12. Complications ensue

I mentioned COVID a while back. I'm not going to get into the full detail of a secondary procedure of the sternotomy I had while I was having my surgery but there was a complication connected to the structural integrity of the sternal repair, requiring me to go back to Stanford and go through the ER. They said, come through the ER, it'll be a little bit easier, it'll be a lot faster, right? This is two weeks out from surgery.

We get there, I'm sitting in the ER, and there's only two or three other people in the entire place. Until I get into the examining room. Now I'm inside the examining room, where there are people in *all* the rooms and there are doctors and nurses flitting back and forth. They get me, they see what the issue was, they fix it, everything's fine. They suggest we're just going to have you stay overnight to be 100% sure all is well. Rather than have you go back tonight, just go back in the morning. So, I do. I get home, and about two days later, I'm now walking outside, I'm taking long walks, feeling really good about myself and feeling good about how things are going. I get this cough, and I don't feel well, and something's not right, and I've got this spirometer that I'm working really, really well, because I think it's important and maybe I can improve my lung capacity by using this device. I'm actually competing with myself on the stupid spirometer. Okay, that was good. Do a little bit better.

But I don't feel well, and I start coughing. Coughing after having had your entire chest opened up means I've become intimate with my red heart pillow. I'm hugging the pillow every time I cough, which is what you're supposed to do to laugh, cough, whatever. Squeeze the pillow tight to your chest. For 24 hours straight, I coughed. I thought that was going to kill me and if not, certainly ruin my sternotomy. Non-stop, 24 hours. The pins are going to come apart. I can't believe this is happening. Of course I couldn't sleep. I'm still downstairs on the couch and I go through this horrific sweating and feverish period and all I can think of is I've got to keep walking. Maybe I had better test for COVID because I feel like crap. But I can't stop walking. I tested positive and next thing you know, of course, my wife the next day has it. It took three days of testing to get a positive result but we knew we had it. The first day we tested, nothing. Second day, uh oh, I got it. Third day, she has it. Hers wasn't quite as severe, but I kept walking. It's important to understand, it's going to be uncomfortable, but you're either walking or resting so unless you're really physically disabled by it all, or not in good enough shape for whatever reason, keep doing what you need to do to heal well. Of course, use common sense and check with your doctor to be sure whatever you're doing is safe.

13. Mind Fullness

The other part of the healing process that is really critical is keeping your mind active as well as your body. Challenge your mind. Be creative. Do something you haven't done before or maybe in a long time. Learn an instrument. Listen to music you've not listened to for a while, read, take up a hobby that's not physically demanding. Engage your mind. Maybe you can do some volunteer work.

Getting out of your head and into somebody else's heart is a great motivator for well-being. Don't just sit on the couch feeling sorry for yourself. Be grateful. You have to stimulate your mind, distract yourself from the pain and discomfort. I truly believe things happen *for* us, not *to* us. How could this have happened for you? What can you do with your life now that you've been given this second chance? What does life look like going forward? Share it with friends and family. Write down some goals or things you've always wanted to do. Play video games. The list goes on and on… just be sure to engage and stimulate your mind.

And more, keep a positive mindset, a positive attitude. You have to have the outlook that this is going to get better, it's going to improve. I'm going to be better. You may not alleviate the symptoms that you had the surgery for completely, but the majority of people are going to have an improved quality of life if they do what they need to do to improve the quality of their life. The surgery is only the beginning.

In the long run, this may even mean changing your circle of friends. You need to take care of you and if you weren't thrilled with your lifestyle before the surgery, now's your chance to make that change. If it means better eating, less drinking, more people with a positive outlook, then find those people you can now relate to and take the support they provide. None of us is capable of doing this alone. We need to share our experiences and stay close to those who support us to be the best version of ourselves we can now be. Falling back on bad habits, even with a repaired bridge, is not going to get you the lifestyle you had hoped to experience without you making some changes.

14. Healing is personal.

So here we are now about three months out. You should be in touch with your thoracic surgeon as well as your cardiac surgeon and everybody's keeping an eye on you and you're talking to them—and if you have any questions, be sure to ask because they may be critical. Everything isn't perfect for everybody.

You also need to know that healing doesn't go the same way for everyone. It's not necessarily linear; it's a trend line, but every day isn't up and there are certainly setbacks. The process is not overnight. *Think over time, not overnight.* Everything will pass. You'll get better and better and better.

And so, as the first month passes, you start to think about, okay, I'm walking, I'm feeling good, I can get out, I can go to the mall, I can go shopping. I can't lift anything yet, but I can travel with my wife. By the second month, you're thinking I could drive. But you can't. They don't want something to happen. So don't. An accident could be dreadful. Not to mention, you may not be quite as astute and aware and reactive. Driving requires you to lift a leg to put a brake on. That's a stomach muscle. You just may not have the strength you need yet so why risk anything? I did cheat and drove a little sooner only to realize you can't get hand over hand on the steering wheel with the sternotomy. Duh.

You're likely going to get referred to cardiac rehab. This is one space I can't offer much detail as I didn't go through any formalized program post-surgery. I don't even know why. I do know the majority of you will go through the process and it's a good one as it builds confidence in your capability under the guidance of medical professionals. They'll monitor your progress every step of the way to insure you don't overdo it and to be certain there are no issues with your heart. I strongly encourage you to explore your options here and do it.

15. Go for a Spin?

Then there was, for me, that first bike ride. As you can imagine, all the while I'm walking, I can't wait to find out when I can get on my bike. Once the cone of sternal protection was lifted at about 12 weeks, I was all over my thoracic surgeon and my cardiologist to see when I could begin the process of getting back into shape on two wheels. For me, the epitome of the healing process would be I could get on my bicycle. My thoracic doc says you can get on the bike, but you can't ride the bike, do you have a stationary situation? You bet. I have it set up in the garage on a rig that lets you just pedal going nowhere. He said, "I'm good with that." He just didn't want me to fall as that could damage something in the sternum. My cardiac surgeon said to be careful, get your cardio up and be comfortable with what's going on with your heart. Give it all a month stationary and then do whatever you want to do depending on how you feel.

YEAH! I get in the garage and I remember I've got my riding gear on and oddly going nowhere. I remember I did an Instagram post of getting on the bicycle, which was not as easy as I thought. It was actually hard. Once I got up there and got my arms on the bars and thought, okay, how does this feel? Everything feels good. Now that the structural part was comfortable and I was aware of what I was going to feel, I now had the cardiac part of it, the real part, the part to be concerned about.

I start pedaling and I've got a heart monitor on, I'm watching everything. Just to be able to do that was a very emotional moment because I was coming back and on the bike. I was toasted after five miles having done really nothing. Five miles is nothing for me and the resistance was set for an easy spin. There was no pressure, I was just happy to have done it. Then I did it again the next day. Thought my legs were going to explode. It was brutal. But just like any exercise, you work back into it and eventually I was back riding as if nothing had ever happened.

That was my cardiac rehab in a sense. There was one frightening experience I'll share simply because it's a part of the process. Now that I knew that my heart was okay from riding on the stationary trainer, it was time to get out on the actual road for a real-world experience.

On road bikes, which is what mine is, we use pedals that your feet are clipped into. You have to move them a particular twisting motion to "unlock" them from the pedal. If you don't, you can't put your leg down to hold yourself up and you fall. Clipping in and taking off for the first ride was a scary experience knowing that if I fell, it could be really painful and worse yet, might even do some real damage. It took a while to get over that anxiety. Again, the range of emotion we get to experience makes us more aware of the significance of what's happened for us. How that is, is up to us.

I'm happy to say, everything went well on those first few rides and I've been riding ever since. Knowing you're reading this after some of the chapters that address my riding efforts, you've now got the full 360 of steps it took to get there.

The same can be true for you whatever it is you choose to set your goals for. Most importantly, do set a goal and continue to strive to work toward it. If it takes 3 months, fine. 6 months, fine. A year, fine. As long as you're making progress and there are no literal health reasons you shouldn't be doing what you're doing, keep inching long, making progress. Your body will thank you. Your mind will thank you and those around you will be thrilled.

CHAPTER 10

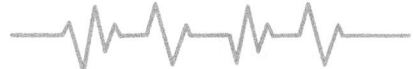

25 Myths and Misconceptions of Myocardial Bridges

WHAT FOLLOWS IS AN OVERVIEW OF THE MANY MYTHS AND MISconceptions about myocardial bridges. Some have already been covered in preceding chapters; however, there are others that just didn't warrant full explanations. I encourage you to continue your journey of education by following some of the direction given earlier in the book if you're interested in learning more about any of the myths and misconceptions below or that you're surely to hear along the way.

A **myocardial bridge (MB)** is a congenital condition where a segment of a coronary artery (most commonly the left anterior descending artery, or LAD) runs through the heart muscle (myocardium) rather than resting on its surface. While generally benign, MBs have been the subject of many myths and misconceptions. Here are some of the most common ones in no particular order:

1. Myocardial bridges do not cause symptoms or complications.

- Reality:
  This is blatantly incorrect. Myocardial bridges DO cause symptoms and complications. While most people with MBs are asymptomatic and lead normal lives, symptoms (such as chest pain, arrhythmias, or even ischemia) do occur in other cases, and while we don't understand why, it's important to note that this could impacting a much greater percentage of the population than previously known.

2. All myocardial bridges require treatment.

- Reality:
  Treatment is typically only necessary for symptomatic cases. Options range from medications (e.g., beta-blockers or calcium channel blockers) to surgical interventions.

3. Myocardial bridges are rare.

- Reality:
  MBs are more common than previously thought. Studies estimate their prevalence at 25-30% in the general population, often identified during autopsies or advanced imaging studies. The estimated percentage of those that become symptomatic is not known.

4. MBs are only diagnosed in adults.

- Reality:
  Myocardial bridges are congenital, meaning they are present from birth. However, they may go undiagnosed until adulthood due to the absence of symptoms or incidental findings during medical imaging. Unfortunately, there are cases of sudden cardiac death in teens as a result of a myocardial bridge.

5. Myocardial bridges may lead to heart attacks.

- Reality:
  While MBs can occasionally contribute to ischemia or myocardial infarction, this typically involves additional factors like atherosclerosis, vasospasm, or the severity of the bridge. Some of those complications, however, could be a direct result of the bridge over time. So, yes, a myocardial bridge can and does cause heart attacks.

6. Exercise is dangerous for people with myocardial bridges.

- Reality:
  For most people with MBs, regular exercise is not harmful and may be encouraged. However, those with symptomatic MBs should consult their healthcare provider to develop a safe exercise plan. In many cases, the bridge is revealed as a result of exertion or exercise and eventually may lead to not only diminished exercise but a complete inability to do so.

7. Myocardial bridges are easily detectable with routine tests.

- Reality:
  This is an absolute falsehood. MBs are often missed during standard coronary angiography because the compression is dynamic, occurring during systole. Advanced imaging techniques, like intravascular ultrasound (IVUS), CT angiography and provocative testing are more reliable yet still need to be addressed by experienced medical professionals.

8. Myocardial bridges worsen with age.

- Reality:
The condition itself doesn't necessarily worsen with age. The consequences, however, most certainly do. This could be as a result of age-related factors like atherosclerosis or simply the constant compression of the artery that causes it to deteriorate. Typically, once symptoms present, they will continue to increase in frequency and severity.

9. Surgery for MB is always the best solution.

- Reality:
Surgery, such as myotomy (cutting the bridge), is reserved for the most symptomatic cases. Many patients respond well to non-surgical treatments like medications or lifestyle changes. Ultimately, surgery may be required as medication does not rectify the root cause of the symptom. It only relieves the discomfort of pain.

10. Myocardial bridges are the sole cause of symptoms that appear to be heart related.

- Reality:
Symptoms like chest pain or palpitations may have multiple causes. Even in patients with MBs, other conditions such as microvascular dysfunction or vasospasm may contribute. It's always best to continue the testing process, the diagnostic process, to best determine the cause of symptoms as many other conditions could present with similar consequences.

11. Myocardial bridges are a type of heart defect.

- Reality:
  While MBs are congenital (present at birth), they are not considered a defect in the same way as structural heart abnormalities like septal defects. They are more accurately described as an anatomical variation.

12. MBs only affect the left anterior descending (LAD) artery.

- Reality:
  Although the LAD artery is the most commonly affected, MBs can involve other coronary arteries that can create symptoms. It's critically important to identify as many arteries as possible in the diagnosis to determine which may be most relevant and possible to "unroof" or treat surgically when symptoms are present.

13. Symptoms of myocardial bridges are always severe.

- Reality:
  Symptoms can range from mild to severe and vary widely. Many individuals with MBs are asymptomatic or experience mild discomfort, while others might develop angina, arrhythmia, or ischemia under specific conditions up to and including debilitating consequences.

14. Coronary stents are one option for myocardial bridges.

- Reality:
  Stents are not the preferred treatment for MBs for many reasons with the primary being that the stent itself cannot withstand the constant compression of the artery and eventually fails, creating an even greater health risk to the patient.

15. Myocardial bridges are static abnormalities.

- Reality:
  No, they are not. MBs cause **dynamic compression** of the artery during the heart's contraction (systole). This distinguishes them from static narrowing like atherosclerosis, where the obstruction is present all the time. This is also what complicates proper diagnosis.

16. A normal stress test rules out MB.

- Reality:
  Unfortunately, it doesn't. A stress test rarely reveals issues caused by MBs, especially in mild cases. How and when symptoms present cannot be pre-determined and re-creating them with a stress test is infrequent at best. Imaging studies like CT angiography or intravascular ultrasound are more definitive with the most detailed being the provocative test.

17. MBs protect against coronary artery disease (CAD).

- Reality:
  There's a misconception that MBs may "shield" the artery segment from developing atherosclerosis. While the tunneled segment may indeed have some protection, the segments before and after the bridge are often more prone to plaque formation due to altered blood flow dynamics. So, in fact, the bridge actually may cause coronary artery disease.

18. Myocardial bridges can "resolve" on their own.

- Reality:
  Never. MBs are congenital and do not "go away." They do not heal.

MYTHS AND MISCONCEPTIONS

19. MBs can only cause symptoms during exertion.

- Reality:
  While exertion can exacerbate symptoms due to increased heart rate and contractility, many symptomatic individuals experience symptoms even at rest, possibly due to coronary vasospasm or other underlying conditions.

20. All chest pain in individuals with MBs is due to the bridge.

- Reality:
  Not all chest pain is related to MBs. Other conditions, such as gastroesophageal reflux disease (GERD), costochondritis, or anxiety, can also cause chest discomfort and need to be ruled out.

21. Myocardial bridges always affect life expectancy.

- Reality:
  For the majority of people, MBs have no significant impact on life expectancy. Symptomatic cases with proper management can mitigate risks and result in comparable life expectancy as someone without a bridge, assuming all things being equal.

22. MBs are unrelated to other heart conditions.

- Reality:
  MBs can coexist with or exacerbate other heart conditions, such as coronary artery disease, vasospastic angina, endothelial dysfunction or hypertrophic cardiomyopathy (HCM).

23. Everyone with a myocardial bridge needs to avoid caffeine or stimulants.

- Reality:
  While stimulants can exacerbate symptoms in sensitive individuals, many people with MBs tolerate moderate caffeine intake. A personalized approach based on symptom triggers is essential.

24. All myocardial bridges are the same.

- Reality:
  MBs vary widely in their characteristics, including depth, length, and severity of arterial compression. These factors however, are unique to each case and are not the leading indication of the severity of the symptoms. Severe symptoms in one individual could be caused by a short, shallow bridge, while a person may be asymptomatic while having a longer, deeper bridge. Each case is unique to the individual.

25. MB symptoms are always due to mechanical compression.

- Reality:
  While systolic compression of the artery is a hallmark of MBs, symptoms can also result from related factors such as endothelial dysfunction, coronary spasm, or abnormal shear stress. Other complications such as atherosclerosis are quite common and while they may ultimately be the result of the bridge, they aren't necessarily always related to the mechanical compression of an artery.

Takeaway

Myths and misconceptions about myocardial bridges can lead to unnecessary anxiety, misdiagnosis, or overtreatment. If you suspect you have or are diagnosed with an MB, consult a cardiologist familiar with this condition for accurate diagnosis and appropriate tailored management.

Glossary of Terms Related to Myocardial Bridges

A

- **Acetylcholine Challenge Test**: A diagnostic test where acetylcholine, a chemical that affects blood vessel function, is injected to provoke coronary artery spasms. This test can help identify endothelial dysfunction or vasospasms in patients with myocardial bridges.
- **Angina**: Chest pain or discomfort caused by reduced blood flow to the heart muscle, common in myocardial bridge patients.
- **Angiogram**: An imaging test that uses X-rays and contrast dye to visualize the coronary arteries and detect abnormalities like myocardial bridges.
- **Aorta**: The largest artery in the body, responsible for carrying oxygenated blood from the heart to the rest of the body.
- **Atherosclerosis**: A condition characterized by plaque buildup inside the arteries, sometimes coexisting with myocardial bridges.
- **ANOCA (Angina with Non-Obstructive Coronary Arteries)**: A condition where patients experience angina despite having no significant blockages in the coronary arteries. Myocardial bridges may be a contributing factor.
- **Anomalous Aortic Origin of a Coronary Artery (AAOCA)**: A rare congenital condition where a coronary artery arises from an abnormal location on the aorta, which can affect blood flow and sometimes coexist with myocardial bridges.

- **Atrium:** One of the two upper chambers of the heart that receives blood returning to the heart from the body or lungs.

B

- **Balloon Angioplasty:** A procedure where a small balloon is inflated inside an artery to open it, sometimes considered when myocardial bridges coexist with other blockages.
- **Beta-Blockers:** Medications that reduce heart rate and blood pressure, often used to manage myocardial bridge symptoms.
- **Blood Pressure:** The force exerted by circulating blood on the walls of blood vessels, which can be influenced by myocardial bridges and related cardiovascular conditions.
- **Bridging Segment:** The portion of the coronary artery that tunnels beneath the heart muscle in myocardial bridges.

C

- **CABG (Coronary Artery Bypass Grafting) Procedure:** A surgical procedure that reroutes blood around a blocked or narrowed coronary artery, occasionally performed in conjunction with unroofing for myocardial bridges.
- **Calcium Channel Blockers:** Medications that relax blood vessels and improve blood flow, often used to manage chest pain in myocardial bridge patients.
- **Cardiac Catheterization:** A procedure in which a catheter is inserted into the heart's blood vessels to measure pressures or inject contrast dye for imaging.
- **Cardiac CT Angiogram (CTA):** A non-invasive imaging test that uses computed tomography and contrast dye to create detailed 3D images of the coronary arteries. It's particularly useful for identifying myocardial bridges and assessing their severity.

GLOSSARY

- **Cardiomyopathy**: A disease of the heart muscle that affects its ability to pump blood effectively. Myocardial bridges can sometimes be associated with hypertrophic cardiomyopathy.
- **Cholesterol**: A waxy, fat-like substance found in the blood. High levels of cholesterol, particularly LDL, can contribute to cardiovascular problems and exacerbate conditions like myocardial bridges.
- **Compression**: The squeezing of a coronary artery by overlying heart muscle, a defining feature of myocardial bridges.
- **Coronary Artery**: The blood vessels that supply oxygenated blood to the heart muscle, including arteries that may be affected by myocardial bridges.

D

- **Diabetes**: A chronic condition characterized by high blood sugar levels that can contribute to endothelial dysfunction and exacerbate symptoms in myocardial bridge patients.
- **Diastole**: The phase of the heartbeat when the heart muscle relaxes and the coronary arteries fill with blood. Myocardial bridges often restrict blood flow during this phase.
- **Diastolic Fractional Flow Reserve**: A specific measurement of blood flow during the diastolic phase, used to assess the impact of myocardial bridges on coronary circulation.
- **Dobutamine Stress Test**: A diagnostic test where dobutamine, a medication that mimics exercise by increasing heart rate and contractility, is used to evaluate myocardial bridges under stress conditions. It helps identify ischemia or other functional effects.
- **Dynamic Compression**: The periodic squeezing of a coronary artery during each heartbeat, often observed in myocardial bridges.
- **Dyspnea**: Shortness of breath, which can be a symptom experienced by patients with myocardial bridges.

GLOSSARY

E

- **Electrocardiogram (ECG or EKG):** A test that records the electrical activity of the heart to identify irregularities, including those caused by myocardial bridges.
- **Endothelial Dysfunction:** A condition where the inner lining of blood vessels doesn't function properly, contributing to symptoms in myocardial bridge patients.

F

- **Fractional Flow Reserve (FFR):** A measurement taken during cardiac catheterization to assess the impact of a myocardial bridge on blood flow through a coronary artery.
- **Instantaneous Wave-Free Ratio (iFR):** A non-invasive, pressure-based measurement taken during cardiac catheterization to evaluate blood flow and the physiological impact of a myocardial bridge without the need for medication-induced stress.

G

- **GERD (Gastroesophageal Reflux Disease):** A digestive disorder that causes acid reflux and heartburn, which can mimic or exacerbate chest pain in myocardial bridge patients.

H

- **Halo:** A radiological finding or artifact seen around a coronary artery, often associated with myocardial bridges.
- **Hemodynamics:** The study of blood flow and pressure within the heart and vessels, often used to assess the impact of myocardial bridges.

- **HDL (High-Density Lipoprotein)**: Often referred to as "good cholesterol," HDL helps remove other forms of cholesterol from the bloodstream, promoting cardiovascular health.
- **Hypertrophic Cardiomyopathy**: A condition where the heart muscle becomes abnormally thick, potentially worsening the effects of myocardial bridges.

I

- **INOCA (Ischemia with Non-Obstructive Coronary Arteries)**: A condition where patients experience ischemia despite having no significant blockages in the coronary arteries. Myocardial bridges and microvascular dysfunction can be contributing factors.
- **Intramyocardial Artery**: A coronary artery that lies embedded within the heart muscle, as seen in myocardial bridges.
- **Ischemia**: Insufficient blood flow to the heart muscle, which can result from the compression caused by a myocardial bridge.
- **Intravascular Ultrasound (IVUS)**: A specialized imaging technique that uses a catheter to visualize the inside of coronary arteries, providing detailed views of myocardial bridges.

L

- **LCX (Left Circumflex Artery)**: A coronary artery that supplies blood to the left side of the heart. It can be affected by myocardial bridges.
- **LDL (Low-Density Lipoprotein)**: Often referred to as "bad cholesterol," LDL contributes to plaque buildup in arteries and increases the risk of heart disease.
- **Life Vest**: A wearable defibrillator designed to monitor heart rhythms and deliver a shock if a life-threatening arrhythmia is detected. While not directly related to myocardial bridges, it may be considered for patients at risk of sudden cardiac arrest due to other underlying conditions.

- **Lipids**: Fats and fat-like substances, including cholesterol and triglycerides, that are important for body functions but can contribute to cardiovascular disease if levels are too high.

M

- **Microvascular Angina**: Chest pain caused by issues in the small blood vessels of the heart, sometimes seen alongside myocardial bridges.
- **MVD (Microvascular Dysfunction)**: A condition where small blood vessels in the heart fail to dilate properly, contributing to chest pain or ischemia, and sometimes co-occurring with myocardial bridges.
- **Milking Effect**: A term used to describe the visible narrowing of a coronary artery during systole due to the compression caused by a myocardial bridge.
- **Minimally Invasive Unroofing Procedure**: A less invasive surgical technique for treating myocardial bridges, typically using smaller incisions on the side and accessing the heart between the ribs.
- **Myocardial Bridge**: A condition in which a coronary artery tunnels through the heart muscle instead of lying on its surface, causing compression during each heartbeat.
- **Myocardium**: The muscular tissue of the heart, involved in myocardial bridges when it compresses an artery.
- **Myotomy**: A surgical procedure to cut muscle fibers, often performed to relieve compression in myocardial bridges.

O

- **Occlusion**: A blockage or closure of a blood vessel, which can occur in coronary arteries and exacerbate conditions like myocardial bridges.

P

- **PAC (Premature Atrial Contraction):** An irregular heartbeat that originates in the atria. While not specific to myocardial bridges, it may occur in patients with heart-related issues.
- **Patient Advocacy:** Efforts by patients or their advocates to raise awareness, seek diagnoses, and push for treatments for conditions like myocardial bridges.
- **Percutaneous Coronary Intervention (PCI):** A non-surgical procedure, such as stenting, used to open narrowed arteries.
- **Plaque:** Fatty deposits that can build up inside arteries, contributing to atherosclerosis.
- **PVC (Premature Ventricular Contraction):** An irregular heartbeat that originates in the ventricles, sometimes associated with heart conditions.
- **Provocative Testing:** Diagnostic tests that intentionally trigger symptoms or abnormalities (e.g., using medications like acetylcholine) to identify underlying conditions such as vasospasms or ischemia caused by myocardial bridges.
- **Prinzmetal's Disease:** A condition characterized by coronary artery spasms, which can mimic or exacerbate symptoms of myocardial bridges.

R

- **Right Coronary Artery (RCA):** A major coronary artery that supplies blood to the right side of the heart, which can also be affected by myocardial bridges.
- **Robotically Assisted Unroofing Procedure:** A minimally invasive surgical technique for unroofing myocardial bridges using robotic assistance to improve precision and recovery time.

GLOSSARY

S

- **Septal Buckling**: A phenomenon where the septum (wall between the heart's chambers) appears distorted due to abnormal forces, often related to myocardial bridges.
- **Septal Coronary Arteries**: Small arteries that branch off the main coronary arteries and supply blood to the heart's septum. These may be affected by myocardial bridges.
- **Sternotomy**: A surgical procedure that involves making an incision down the middle of the sternum allowing access to the heart, often used in traditional unroofing surgery.
- **Stenosis**: A narrowing of the coronary arteries that can reduce blood flow, sometimes coexisting with myocardial bridges.
- **Stent**: A small, mesh-like tube inserted into a coronary artery to keep it open.
- **Stress Test**: A diagnostic test to evaluate how the heart performs under physical or pharmacological stress, often used to assess the symptoms of myocardial bridges.
- **Systole**: The phase of the heartbeat when the heart muscle contracts, compressing a tunneled artery in myocardial bridges.

T

- **Tachycardia**: An abnormally fast heart rate, which may exacerbate symptoms in myocardial bridge patients or be a secondary issue.
- **Target Heart Rate**: The heart rate range used during a stress test to evaluate symptoms related to myocardial bridges.
- **Thoracotomy**: A surgical procedure involving an incision into the chest wall between the ribs, to access the heart or lungs, occasionally used for myocardial bridge-related surgeries.

- **Transesophageal Echocardiogram (TEE):** A specialized echocardiogram where a probe is inserted into the esophagus to get clearer images of the heart.
- **Tunneled Artery:** Another term for a myocardial bridge, where a segment of the coronary artery is embedded in the heart muscle.

U

- **Unroofing Surgery:** A definitive surgical treatment for myocardial bridges, where the overlying heart muscle is removed to relieve artery compression.

V

- **Vascular Stiffness:** The loss of elasticity in blood vessels, which can compound issues in myocardial bridge patients.
- **Vasospasm:** Sudden constriction of a coronary artery, which can mimic or worsen symptoms caused by myocardial bridges.
- **Ventricle:** One of the two lower chambers of the heart responsible for pumping blood out to the body or lungs.

This glossary provides an overview of the many of the key terms related to myocardial bridges, including diagnostic methods, treatments, and symptoms. It is intended to serve as a reference only for understanding this condition and its impact. It should not be used in lieu of formal medical advice from a medical professional.

PHOTO PAGES DESCRIPTIONS:

PHOTO PAGE 1—Left to Right

(Top row)
-The Markleeville fire that broke out the day before the Death Ride that may have saved my life. And we thought it might just blow out and we would carry on. What were we thinking!
-My first meeting with Dr. Rishi Menon as a guest on one of our productions in studio. Who knew was about to be my new best friend? This was August 25, 2021.
-My second meeting with Dr. Rishi Menon, now my new best friend the very next day as I had my heart attack on August 26th, 2021. This is where you become a believer in divine inspiration.
-Don't you just love the fashion statement a "life vest" makes?

(Middle row)
-What a pain in the neck. This is how they get everything into you, mainline, post-surgery.
-A great way to lose weight and conditioning. Pre-surgery, 150lbs of me, post-surgery, 138 lbs. Same as high school.
-Let's get scrubbed up and ready for surgery! Hangin' in the hall with Dr. Kumran Mangalam from India prior to joining Dr. Husam Balkhy in the OR to witness a robotic unroofing procedure. It was beyond my wildest dreams. Best part is I now have a wonderful relationship with the patient as well.
-Dr. Husam Balkhy at the helm of the controls for the Da Vinci SI robot as he performs the surgery. He's all hands and feet!

(Bottom row)
-That's my original chest pre-surgery.
-Clearly, my chest post-surgery shortly after the wax had been removed. The drain tube holes are covered to prevent infection.
-Healing nicely, about 4 months out. Notice those drainage tube holes. Wow! I should have drawn a smiley face.
-About 18 months out. Back in the gym and all is good. No, it wasn't easy.

PHOTO PAGE 1

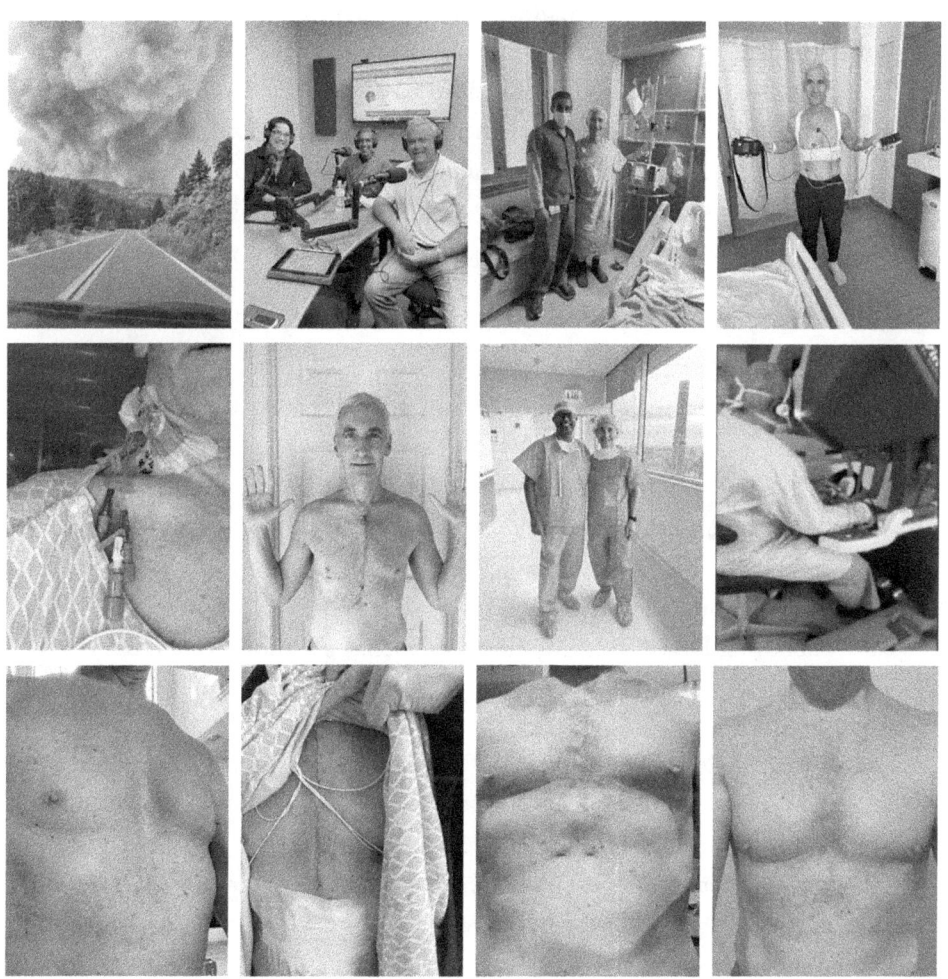

PHOTO PAGES DESCRIPTIONS:

PHOTO PAGE 2—Left to Right

(Top row)
-Yay! Let's go home. Don't do as I did. You're supposed to sit in the back seat.
-Home at last. Only one week prior to getting Covid. I look so comfortable, don't I?
-The rig to sleep sitting up. Seriously. I added a heating pad too.
-That's what the now outdated Da Vinci SI machine looks like. This machine is extinct. Intuitive Surgical, the manufacturer, has not replaced the valued and necessary stabilizer on the newer XI machine. The stabilizer makes for a simpler process to complete the surgery. They won't answer my questions as to why.

(Middle row)
-Dr. Mangalam, Dr. Balkhy and yours truly at University of Chicago Medical Center.
-The wonderful woman who really got the recognition of myocardial bridges started, Dr. Ingela Schnittger.
-A meeting with Sarah Miller and Veronica Thaxton while we all were in Northern California.
-Yes, about that Death Ride. My finish in 2023. I got the ice cream baby!

(Bottom row)
-Sarah Miller, Amanda Pearlman and me. Coffee for three. We live in a ten mile radius of each other. How cool is that?
-Celebrating a ride on my third anniversary of surgery, January 4th, 2025.
-The group photo of those who attended the first ever myocardial bridge meetup, September 2024. It was incredible.

PHOTO PAGE 2

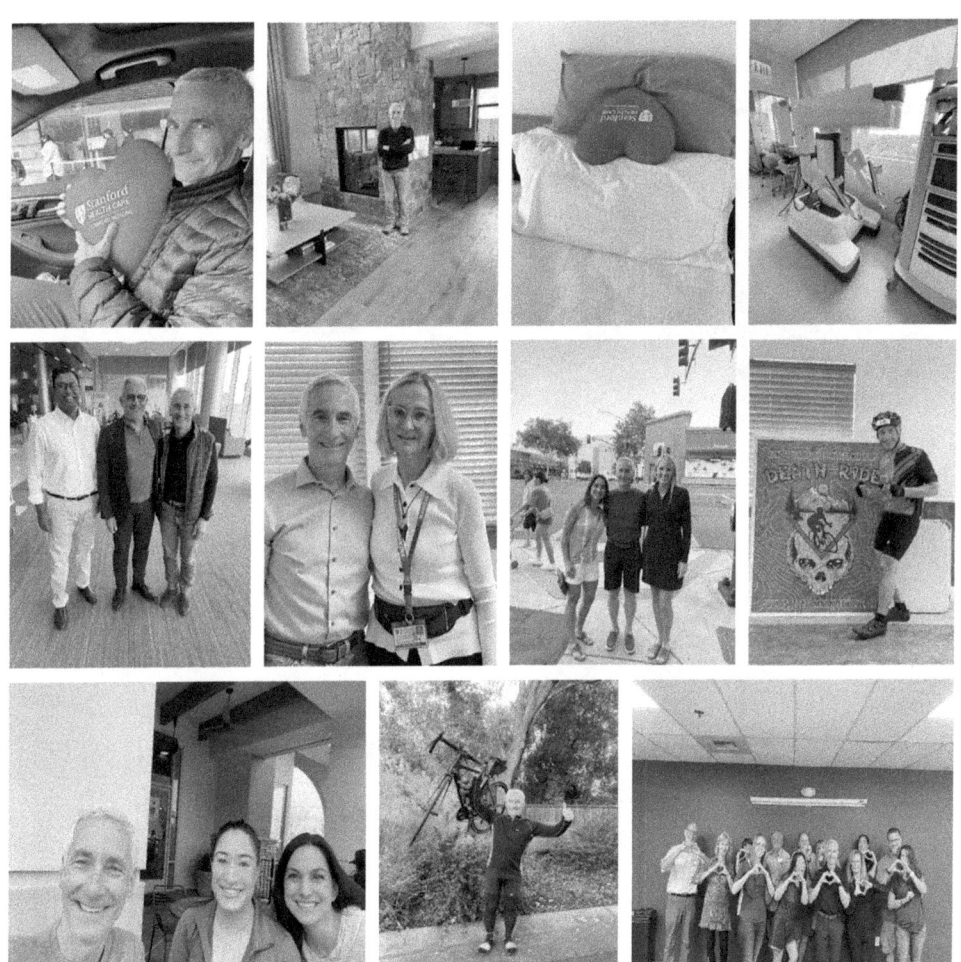

Medical Disclaimer and Release of Liability

This book is intended for informational and educational purposes only and is not a substitute for professional medical advice, diagnosis, or treatment. The content, including comments, statements, personal experiences, and stories provided by both individuals with a myocardial bridge as well as medical professionals, reflects their individual perspectives and experiences. It should not be interpreted as universal medical advice or guidance applicable to all individuals.

Readers are strongly advised to consult a qualified and licensed healthcare provider for any concerns related to myocardial bridges or other medical conditions. The information in this book is not intended to establish a doctor-patient relationship or to provide specific treatment recommendations.

Release of Liability

The author, publisher, and contributors to this book, including medical professionals who have shared their stories or opinions, are released from all liability for any direct, indirect, or consequential damages arising from the use, application, or interpretation of the information contained herein. This includes, but is not limited to:

- Misinterpretation or misuse of the information presented.
- Decisions made by readers regarding their health or medical care.

- Outcomes resulting from actions taken or not taken based on the book's content.

The medical professionals contributing to this book have shared their personal experiences and professional insights for informational purposes only. Their contributions do not constitute medical advice, nor should they be considered endorsements of specific treatments, procedures, or diagnostic methods.

By reading this book, you acknowledge that:

1. The information provided is not a substitute for consulting your healthcare provider.
2. You assume full responsibility for any actions or decisions you make based on the content of this book.
3. You release the author, publisher, and contributors from any liability, claims, or damages, whether known or unknown, arising from your use of this book.

If you are experiencing a medical emergency or have specific health concerns, please contact a licensed healthcare professional immediately.

About the Author

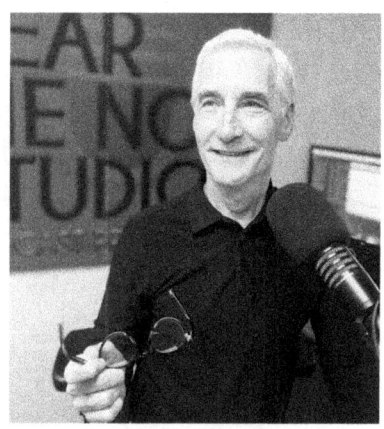

Broadcast pro turned podcast leader, Jeff Holden, made the successful leap from analog to digital audio in 2013 founding NewSense Strategies, Inc. dba Hear Me Now Studio. Under his leadership, these ventures have flourished, producing dozens of shows, increasing brand awareness and financial growth for his clients through authentic storytelling and coaching to directly target each company's specific niche market. Included in those programs are the award winning "Financial Sobriety" now rebranded as "The Whole Wealth Journey" podcast and his own niche health podcast "Imperfect Heart". Driven by his passion to serve, Jeff also launched "The Non Profit Podcast Network" aiming to revolutionize the way non-profit organizations communicate their stories.

A seasoned broadcast professional with over 35 years of successful experience growing audience and revenue, he embarked on his journey in Chicago before making significant contributions in Dallas and ultimately settling in Sacramento, California in 1985. Throughout his career, he has demonstrated a skill for sales and general management, operating local radio stations as well as national sales offices and launching multiple stations across diverse formats including Spanish and Urban.

As the former Central California Regional VP and General Manager of iHeartRadio's multi-station cluster in Sacramento, Jeff played a pivotal role in the sustained success of KFBK AM/FM, one of the nation's oldest and most influential news/talk stations.

Beyond his entrepreneurial pursuits, he remains deeply engaged in the Sacramento community, serving on the Capital Public Radio board and lending his expertise to various non-profit initiatives. With an unwavering commitment to innovation and storytelling, he continues to shape the landscape of broadcasting and podcasting alike. He and his wife have four grown children and twin granddaughters. He's an avid cyclist and automotive enthusiast and loves listening to, well…podcasts.

Life Unfolds For Us

Through trials faced and lessons learned,
In every twist, each page we've turned,
The path was made, the steps aligned,
Not just by fate, but by design.
The storms we feared, the nights so long,
All shaped our hearts and made us strong.
Not *to* us did troubles fall,
But *for* us, our growth, to heed the call.
Healing comes, though not in flight,
But over time, not overnight.
Each scar a map, each tear a sign,
That strength is built in life's design.
With gratitude, I rise today,
For lessons learned along the way.
The highs, the lows, the in-between,
Each moment shaping what has been.
For every gift, for light divine,
For guiding love through space and time,
I lift my heart, my thanks to Thee,
Oh God, who walks this path with me.
So here we stand, with hearts made new,
Embracing all life leads us through.
For every challenge, every mile,
Has led us here, to love, to smile.

JH

www.ingramcontent.com/pod-product-compliance
Lightning Source LLC
Chambersburg PA
CBHW062112040426
42337CB00043B/3727